Neur

FOOD FOR FLOURISHING

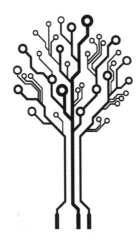

Richard Chalon Aiken MD PhD

Go Ahead Publishing

Los Angeles, California

Go Ahead Publishing
Los Angeles, California

www.goaheadpublishing.com

Neurodietetics/ Richard Chalon Aiken, M.D., Ph.D. —1st ed.

ISBN-13: 978-0692797280

Dedication

This book is dedicated to the millions of people who now or in the future needlessly suffer from cognitive, emotional, or behavioral disorders in part as a result of their dietary patterns. May you heal and flourish.

Contents

Dedication...iii

List of Figures xvii

Preface xix

    Scope of the problem...xix

    How to read this book.. xx

Part I WHEN

CHAPTER 1...25

Evolution and Mental Desolation.....................................25

    Did Gronk see a zombie? 25

    The first psychiatric post-mortem of man....................27

    The dawn of mental disorders 29

    Psychological emergence of mental disorders 31

    Diagnostic classification and evolutionary psychiatry ..32

    Schizophrenia 33

CHAPTER 2...37

Historical Perspective on Mood and Food 37

    Introduction...37

    Trepanation 38

Earliest historical records of mood disorder 38

Ayurveda 40

Biblical.. 41

Hippocrates 42

The medieval period.. 44

The Renaissance 45

The Enlightenment... 45

The modern era.. 46

Recent history of mood disorder prevalence 50

Mood and food 55

Part II WHY

CHAPTER 3 59

Nutritional Programming, Mood through the Lifespan 59

Introduction 59

Adult dietary patterns and mood................................ 60

The Mediterranean diet....................................... 64

Vegetarian diet.. 67

Vegan... 70

Adolescent dietary patterns – junk food, junk moods .. 70

Dietary patterns and depression............................. 75

Fetal 77

Geriatric: The effect of diet on mood and cognition 77

CHAPTER 4 83

Cerebrovascular Disease 83

   Nutrient delivery – the circulatory system 85

   The "Sacred Disease" 87

   Atherosclerosis 91

   Anatomy of cerebrovascular disease 92

   It's the cholesterol 95

   Cerebrovascular disease and depression 97

   Show me the lesion 98

   Different strokes for different folks 100

   "Silent" cerebral infarction and mood 102

   Blood pressure 104

     Not worth our salt 105

   Non-infarction cerebrovascular disease, depression . 105

   Alzheimer's Disease 107

     Genetics 108

     Epidemiology 109

   Vascular disease causes tissue damage 111

   Avoiding saturated fat 111

CHAPTER 5 113

Neuroinflammation 113

  Plants as animals 113

  Plant-based aspirin..................................... 114

  I ignite.. 117

  Epidemiologic evidence relating diet to inflammation 120

  Association of inflammation with depression............. 124

  Dietary interventions for depressive disorders 126

  PUFAs 127

    PUFA sources 132

  Arachidonic acid.. 133

  Stress and inflammation................................. 134

CHAPTER 6 137

Stress 137

  Introduction 137

  The subcellular origin of oxidative stress................... 137

  Taming the fire – the purpose of antioxidants 141

  Physiologic oxidative stress 142

  Food synergy.. 144

  Psychological stress and inflammation..................... 146

  Plant stress response: xenohormesis........................ 149

  Relationship of oxidative stress and inflammation..... 151

Oxidative stress and mental disorders........................152

Neuronal regeneration in the adult............................154

Mitochondrial disorder and mental disorder..............156

CHAPTER 7...157

Gut Feelings 157

The gut-brain axis 157

Psychiatric disorders and the gut-brain axis 160

Attention deficit hyperactivity disorders (ADHD).....163

The intestinal epithelium...163

Leaky gut...164

Psychobiotics..164

Part III WHAT

CHAPTER 8...171

The Science and Art of Nutrition 171

Food as art 171

Neurogastronomy 173

Food as survival..174

Water..177

Magnesium..178

Lithium..180

Dehydration 182

Macronutrients 183

CHAPTER 9 185

Fat 185

   Your fat 185

   Omega-3 fatty acids 186

   The bad fats: Fish oil supplements? 188

   No fish story 189

   DHA 192

   PUFAs in preventing and reversing depression 194

      Building a happier brain: neurogenesis 195

      Omega-6 to omega-3 ratio "6-to-3" 195

   Fat composition 197

      Achieve an adequate omega-3 and 6-to-3 ratio 200

CHAPTER 10 203

Protein 203

   Protein in perspective 203

   How much protein? 205

   Amino acids typical in American diets 207

   Could you be protein deficient? 208

   The optimal protein diet 208

   Do you know beans? 209

   Protein quality 211

Other special protein requirements 212

Life, death, and proteins 213

CHAPTER 11 215

Carbohydrates 215

Our critical energy source 215

Mental effort 217

Desperately seeking fiber 218

CHAPTER 12 221

Macronutrient Distribution 221

Caloric macronutrient distribution 221

The Okinawa traditional diet 223

Energy density versus nutrient density 225

A note on the definition of nutrient density 228

Part IV WHERE

CHAPTER 13 231

Good Mood Food 231

Whole-food varied-plants 231

Cerebrovascular disease 232

Dietary interventions for cerebrovascular disease .. 233

Exercise 241

Stroke 243

Blood pressure and salt 244

Non-Steroidal Anti-Inflammatory Drugs (NSAIDS). 246

Weight.. 246

Habits 247

Psychological stress.. 247

Monitoring 247

Flaxseeds... 248

Hibiscus flowers 249

Just say NO 251

Inflammation.. 254

Fruits and vegetables.. 255

Omega-3 256

Oxidative stress 259

Total antioxidant content...................................... 262

CHAPTER 14 271

Psychotropic Nutraceutics 271

Happy meals 271

Green leafy vegetables 272

Green tea 272

Fruits 276

Nuts and seeds 277

Seeds 278

Whole grain 282

Nutritional yeast.. 285

Cocoa 286

Herbs and spices 287

    Turmeric 288

    Ground peppercorns.................................... 290

    Saffron... 292

    Hibiscus flowers 296

    Rooibos 297

    Rhodiola 299

    Maca root 301

    Ashwagandha roots (withania somnifera)............... 302

Supplements.. 303

    Vitamin B_{12} 303

    Vitamin D.. 304

    Omega-3 supplements 311

    Iodine.. 311

    Sleep supplements 314

    Plant stanols, sterols 315

Part V HOW

CHAPTER 15 319

High Temperature Thermal Processing...................... 319

Thermal processing and antioxidant activity 321

Introduction to other vegetable processing methods . 323

CHAPTER 16 325

Low Temperature Thermal Processing......................... 325

Dehydration... 325

Sous vide 328

Sous vide setup 330

CHAPTER 17 333

Mechanical Processing....................................... 333

Blending: a tornado in the kitchen 333

Bioaccessibility... 335

Blender mechanical properties............................... 336

Oxidation... 337

Freezing greens 341

Crushing: The Stone Age way................................ 344

CHAPTER 18 349

Special Occasions 349

Roasting and cooking over an open fire 349

Sacred four-directions harvest table thanksgiving 349

The celebration...351

CHAPTER 19...355

Changing Habits using Cognitive Behavioral Therapy.. 355

How to change your dietary pattern............................355

What is your why 356

It's the thought that counts......................................356

Cognitive and Behavioral Therapies.......................358

Why use CBT? 359

Socratic questioning...359

The CBT model of the human experience 360

Trigger happy 361

Think again 363

The CBT brain circuit..365

Case Study: Stinkin' Thinkin'.................................365

Defense Mechanisms 367

Denial 368

Rationalization...368

Projection 368

Reaction Formation 368

Regression 369

List of Figures

Figure 1 Mentally Ill Hospitalized Patients 51
Figure 2 Severe Mental Illness 52
Figure 3 Mood Disorder per 1000 53
Figure 4 Omega-3 to Omega-6 Ratio 129
Figure 5 Xenohormesis 149
Figure 6 Fat, Omega-3 and "6 to 3" ratios 199
Figure 7 Essential Amino Acids Daily Requirements 210
Figure 8 The New Ancestral Diet Macronutrient Distribution 222
Figure 9 SAD Macronutrient Composition.............................. 223
Figure 10 The Okinawa Diet Macronutrient Distribution 224
Figure 11 RAM Various Macronutrient Compositions............ 225
Figure 12 Energy Density and Nutrient Density 226
Figure 13 Nutrient Density to Energy Density Ratio.............. 227
Figure 14 Antioxidant Properties of Select Beverages 263
Figure 15 Antioxidant Content of Select Fruits...................... 264
Figure 16 Antioxidant Properties of Select Vegetables 265
Figure 17 Antioxidant Content of Select Nuts and Seeds....... 266
Figure 18 Antioxidant Contents of Select Herbs and Spices... 269
Figure 19 Relative Mortality Risk v. Whole Grain Intake........ 284
Figure 20 Antioxidant Loss from cooking, percent................. 322
Figure 21 Questions that Probe Reason and Evidence........... 360

Preface

Is it a paradox to suggest we need science to achieve a natural state of health? That appears to be precisely our situation – the current trend toward dietary deficiencies amongst abundance is swiftly veering away from our evolutionary survivalist trajectory with dire health consequences – not only involving physical health but mental health as well.

The brain is the most sensitive organ in our body and manifests its pathology cognitively, emotionally, and behaviorally, often insidiously. Diet has a profound influence on our minds. With some understanding of these effects, we can relieve suffering and possibly help reverse neuropsychiatric pathology.

Even without overt clinical signs of physical, cognitive, or emotional decline, we can achieve a profound state of mind-body wellness, eudaimonia — human flourishing — with proper lifestyle choices. This book is about mind-body flourishing through dietary choices that the author calls "neurodietetics."

SCOPE OF THE PROBLEM

In 2014, an estimated 43.6 million adults aged 18 or older in the United States alone had mental illness, according to the National Institute of Mental Health; this number represented 18.1% of all adults. That same source stated that over 20 percent of our children, either currently or at some point during their life, will have a seriously debilitating mental disorder.

According to the World Health Organization, an estimated 350 million people of all ages suffer from depression globally and is the leading cause of disability worldwide.

Even with a growing recognition of this problem and ever more medical interventions, the situation is rapidly getting worse. We are doing something wrong and that something has to do with lifestyle, specifically diet.

HOW TO READ THIS BOOK

My own dietary lifestyle changes happened rather quickly after becoming educated on nutritional medicine, something I did not get in formal medical or scientific training. I am hoping that once you have thorough scientific evidence of how food affects mental wellness, you will make some adjustments accordingly.

This book is divided into five parts. Our approach is reminiscent of Rudyard Kipling's (1865—1936) analysis of a subject employing "six honest men":

> *"I have six honest serving men,*
> *They taught me all I knew.*
> *Their names are What,*
> *and Where and When;*
> *and Why and How and Who."*

The first honest person is you, the *Who*.

- ❖ Part I, *When*, looks at the beginnings of mental illness and what appears to have affected its auspicious meteoric rise.

❖ Part II, *Why*, unabashedly examines the exciting new science behind causation of cognitive and emotional disorders. In this book, I attempt to remove my own personal opinions as much as I can in favor of well-researched facts. In this part, there are a lot of facts with extensive references. Please don't be discouraged by the detail.

❖ Part III, *What*, is an overview on nutrition basics, particularly as it applies to the mind. Think nutrition is all about protein, fat, carbohydrates, and a few vitamins and minerals? Think again.

❖ Part IV, *Where*, is about ideal mood foods, with the reasoning explained. Simple specific suggestions and practical ideas are featured.

❖ Part V, *How*, explains food processing techniques that favor convenience and flavor without compromising or destroying nutrition. It also gives suggestions on how to change eating habits using an evidence - based approach, called cognitive behavioral therapy.

The human condition involves scientific fields pertaining to the biological, the psychological, and the ecological. We might think of this as the body (biological), mind (psychological), and environment (ecological). The environment that directly affects the mind-body of concern here is food.

Should you currently be experiencing physical or mental disorders, please consult an appropriate professional. The ideas in this book are intended to be potentially helpful resources best incorporated into holistic considerations by you and your physician. You may need to provide a copy of this book to your doctor, however, as this material is not yet generally known.

Let us seek eudaimonia in the original Aristotelian sense: well-being as the result of an active life governed by reason. Reason follows.

Part I WHEN

When did disturbances of a neuropsychiatric nature begin? What influenced the emergence of cognitive and emotional problems so frequent in our society today? The answers to these questions have important implications on etiology, prevention, and treatment of the sub-optimal mind-body.

CHAPTER 1

Evolution and Mental Desolation

"Though I shall get more kicks than half-pennies, I will, life serving, attempt my work. "

Charles Darwin

DID GRONK SEE A ZOMBIE?

Imagine the scene of a hominid-ish looking mortal obviously wildly wounded and smelling of rotting flesh staggering his way toward an individual from the mid-Paleolithic Period[1], about 1.5 million years ago. We shall for purposes of argument refer to the rotting man as a "zombie" and the Paleolithic man as "Gronk". The ensuing conversation follows:

---

[1] The Paleolithic Period spanned from 2.5 million years ago to about ten thousand years ago; this roughly also spans the Stone Age, which is estimated to have lasted from 3.5 million years ago to about 5,000 years ago.

Zombie: "oooooo," moaning flatly and repetitiously.

Gronk[2]: "hmmmmm."

Going along with the zombie supposition, zombie's verbal expression might correspond to "meat" as that is the only motivation driving such a beast, at least as folklore would have it. Gronk's response *"hmmmmm"* is also an acronym for "holistic, manipulative, multi-modal, musical, and mimetic[3]," elements of a basic pre-linguistic system used in various forms until roughly 100 thousand years ago when genetic representations of more advanced use of the tongue, lips, and larynx appear[4], allowing more advanced ability to make subtle sound nuances and the likelihood of oral communication. But here Gronk's "hmmmmm" may have been used defensively as a mimetic variation on a growl.

The apparent adversarial nature of this meeting in which zombie advances in the described manner would likely result in Gronk, who was much faster and goal-directed than zombie, running away to safety. Note that Gronk, although living half-way through the Paleolithic Period, would have no weapons – that wouldn't happen for another million to a million and a half years.

Yes, this was also the Stone Age, and although Gronk was familiar with stones for simple food processing such as grinding and stripping-off desirable edible plant parts, he had not yet

---

[2] Gronk is a name assigned in popular literature to a typical man who lived in the Paleolithic Period, so-called "Paleo man".

[3] Mithen, Steven J. (2006). *The singing neanderthals: The origins of music, language, mind, and body.* Cambridge, Mass.: Harvard University Press.

[4] Jakobson, R. and M. Halle 1956. *Fundamentals of Language.* The Hague: Mouton.

regarded stones as weapons other than perhaps for frightening off certain smaller animals from a distance by tossing small stones at them. And he never carried stones around with him.

Nor would Gronk be interested in the zombie as a food source (not even considering its rotting infectious nature). Although there was some degree of opportunistic scavenging of meat much later, about two hundred and fifty thousand years ago, it wasn't until about 40 thousand years ago – or 1.4 % of the Paleolithic Period – that Homo Sapiens could even primitively hunt; and that was merely a supplement to their whole-food varied-plant dietary pattern[5].

THE FIRST PSYCHIATRIC POST-MORTEM OF MAN

Okay first, unless anyone has hard evidence of otherwise, there are no zombies. But let's imagine Gronk holds to the above-described story and communicates (sort of) to his fellow Paleoites. Is he crazy? What other explanation could there be?

This is a more important question than one might think. If Gronk was psychotic, in the modern clinical psychiatric sense, that would establish such illness very early indeed in the history of our species.

Before we delve further into this, I will provide the additional information that Gronk has no history of major medical illnesses, seizures, black-outs or head injuries. He is 18 years old, five feet tall, weighs 125 lbs. and is in excellent physical condition. He lives with about 15 others; he has fathered three children by two different females. His interests include eating, foraging for food, showing his prowess by providing food for "the others" as well as sexual intercourse. He has been

---

[5] Aiken, R.C. and D. Aiken (2015) *The New Ancestral Diet* p 41, Go-Ahead Publishing.

exploring today as always for additional plant sources of food, including roots, seeds, nuts, and leaves.

A claim of a close encounter with a flesh eating zombie could by some standards in some societies be the basis for a diagnosis of a psychotic disorder. In other societies, perhaps this could be considered a visionary experience with religious interpretation.

This is not the case with Gronk for several reasons. First, Gronk had no real language or capacity for rational thought and conceptualization. At his disposal were instinct, sense memories, pattern recognition, very rudimentary forms of intelligence. Without the concept of the past, there were no depressing or terrifying thoughts that would revisit his consciousness; without the concept of the future, there were no fears or anxieties associated with the future.

Now with the added supposition that there never were such creatures as zombies, we must assume that Gronk experienced a psychotic episode. This is peculiar because

- We have no information concerning a similar previous episode.
- He does not appear psychotic otherwise.
- Psychotic disorders 1.5 million years ago would be un- likely, certainly not genetically favored so they would have been eradicated by natural selection.

There couldn't have been severe mental disorders at that time. Not only was Gronk a non-thinking hominid in the true sense but also based on the fact that no genetic material that could lead to one's destruction could be expressed and passed on for thousands of millennia.

Conclusion: Gronk most likely hallucinated after consuming an unknown toxic plant.

Many today have the concept of caveman Gronk that is closer to that of the zombie than individuals who actually lived during the Paleolithic Period at least in regard to their preferred food group. Worse, some modern-day "Paleo" enthusiasts eat meat aimlessly while there is current day understanding that it leads to disease and demise.

THE DAWN OF MENTAL DISORDERS

There are three basic causative factors that can lead to mental disorders: one is of the physical realm and inherent to the individual; let's refer to that as the *body*; the other is the result of processing sensorial information - let's refer to that as the realm of the *mind;* the third is an exterior element – the realm of the environment.

For animals and primitive man, the mind-body connection existed primarily to optimize the likelihood of survival of the organism in order to procreate. They had the abilities of sensation and perception but not that of conceptualization. Sensations are integrated into perceptions automatically. To integrate perceptions into concepts requires a much higher level of consciousness, that of thought: reasoning. Homo sapiens sapiens achieved anatomical modernity[6] about two

---

[6] A number of anatomical changes occurred rather rapidly including lessening of the skeletal strength and corresponding muscle mass; D. Jeffrey Meldrum, Charles E. Hilton. From Biped to Strider: The Emer-

hundred thousand years ago but it does not appear that they had rudiments of modern human behaviors and thus thought, until about fifty thousand years ago[7] after which time technical and artistic artifacts have been found.

Undoubtedly early hominids suffered from a variety of physical ailments of the body, such as infections, injury, and malnutrition/ starvation. Such environmentally imposed insults could directly affect the functioning of their minds – but this is not what we mean today as a mental disorder. Any single definition of mental disorder is not all-inclusive; however, the latest official definition of mental disorder is[8]:

> *"a syndrome characterized by clinically significant disturbance in an individual's (baseline) cognition, emotion regulation, or behavior that reflects a dysfunction in the psychological, biological, or developmental processes underlying mental functioning. Mental disorders are usually associated with significant distress in social, occupational, or other important activities."*

The parenthetical word "baseline" is my addition, as a disorder can only take place if it deviates from the "normal" state of that individual. This is a rather broad definition – it even includes mental and behavioral states that are primarily the result of

---

gence of Modern Human Walking, Running and Resource Transport. Springer, 31 March 2004.

[7] Mellars, Paul (2006). "Why did modern human populations disperse from Africa ca. 60,000 years ago?" Proceedings of the National Academy of Sciences 103 (25):9381 – 6.

[8] American Psychiatric Association. (2013). Diagnostic and statistical manual of mental disorders: DSM-5. Washington, D.C: American Psychiatric Association.

other bodily disease processes such as stroke or dementias. Inherent in this definition is that the individual is capable of conscious cognitive, behavioral and emotional conceptualizations, viz., "modern humans."

Short of actual physical damage from external or internal processes, the environment plays an important role in the emergence of mental disorder. For example, while genetics is a relatively fixed mind-body element, epigenetic influences, emanating from the environment, can determine if a certain combination of genes are switched on or off. We shall explore in detail the genetic, hormonal, neuronal, and immune functions that operate together in a complex way to result in mental health or disorder in Part II.

PSYCHOLOGICAL STRESS AND THE EMERGENCE OF MENTAL DISORDERS

Other than disordered mood states as a direct result of physical processes or disease, invariably there is a significant contribution from psychological stress. These can be quite variable and depend on many factors, including one's conditioned experiential conceptualizations. Resiliency and coping abilities are intertwined with genetic and epigenetic factors affected by imposed environmental conditions as well as lifestyle choices (for example, diet and exercise).

Without the ability to conceptualize, i.e. possess basic abstract thinking, mental disorder as we know it is not possible. The potential gain of being fully conscious, of course, can be an enormous advantage and would have to be recognized as the single most significant result of our evolution as a species.

Therefore, the advantages of intelligence can be a double-edged sword unless we are able to control our thinking. Chapter 19 outlines the state-of-the-art tool, Cognitive

Behavioral Therapy, to assist in making rational choices that benefit one emotionally and behaviorally. The example focus is on making correct dietary choices that lead to optimal mental health rather than pure culinary pleasures.

On the basis of the evolution of conceptualization, there could not have been mental disorders before about fifty thousand years ago

---

So the evolution of mental disorders is a rather recent phenomenon on the evolutionary scale. How recent? Mood disorders do not leave survivable descriptive artifacts until there was written history. Let's look next at that record to understand origins. Doing so will reveal enormous implications.

DIAGNOSTIC CLASSIFICATION AND EVOLUTIONARY PSYCHIATRY

There have been countless historical references to madness, deviance, lunacy, and insanity, but rarely with definitions or classification of signs and symptoms. This is a major problem in the field of psychiatry that we are only recently beginning to understand. There is likely a very broad spectrum of types and subtypes and cross-overs that render any attempt to classify mental disorders very challenging. We shall explore some of the etiologic complexities in Part II that help illustrate the classification of mental disorder dilemma.

Let's take as an example the problem of a specific diagnosis, that of schizophrenia. The account of Pinel[9] in 1809 may be the

---

[9] Pinel, P. (1809). Traité médico-philosophique sur l'aliénation mentale (2nd ed.). Paris: Brosson.

first description that we identify today as being consistent with our general classification of schizophrenia. The first classification of more general mental disorders was that of Kraepelin[10] in 1893, who basically divided mental disorder into affective states and schizophrenia (his terminology for the latter state was Dementia Praecox).

Prior to 1700, cases of "insanity" seldom had reported auditory hallucinations – perhaps the most seminal symptom of the condition termed schizophrenia that we recognize today. Psychosis was apparently relatively brief and often occurred in the presence of other diseases[11]. In fact, epidemiologic evidence supports a very recent increase in the prevalence of this disorder, as we shall explore later.

SCHIZOPHRENIA

Nevertheless, for the sake of illustration let us assume that some form of what we call today the psychiatric disorder "schizophrenia" was present in early Homo sapien sapien times, say sometime after fifty thousand years ago. The enigma is how could such a devastating mental disorder not be "deselected" genetically, as it does not support the continuation of the species.

One of the favorite explanations of this dilemma by evolutionary-inclined psychiatrists is the "balancing selection" theory[12] [13]. In such a scenario, the genes that are conducive to

---

[10] Kraepelin, E. (1893). Psychiatrie: Ein Lehrbuch für Studierende und Ärzte (4th ed.). Leipzig: Barth.

[11] Torrey, E. F., & Miller, J. (2001). The invisible plague: the rise of mental illness from 1750 to the present. New Jersey: Rutgers University Press.

[12] Allen J, Sarich V. Schizophrenia in an evolutionary per- spective. Perspect Biol Med 1988;32:132–53.

schizophrenia are being kept in the human genome because of the unusual advantages they (or their allelic variants) may offer in a different genetic configuration. Such advantages are enjoyed mostly by the close relatives of the schizophrenics rather than the individual with the fully expressed disorder.

The oft-quoted favorite example of balancing selection – they are rare – is that of sickle cell anemia, a disease that is commonly observed in people from African and Mediterranean heritage. Geneticists have shown that anemic patients are (recessively) homozygotic (aa) for b-hemoglobin in their DNA. Dominantly homozygotic (AA) individuals do not develop anemia, but are susceptible to malaria, which have been very common in some parts of Africa and the Mediterranean. Heterozygotics (Aa), however, do not produce anemia and are resistant to malaria. So the net effects of these allelic variants (aa, AA, Aa) "balance" each other in this sense.

That example is used to speculate that close relatives to individuals with schizophrenia seem to have greater creativity (for example, in Albert Einstein's son[14], James Joyce's daughter[15], and Carl Gustav Jung's mother) and individuals with a milder form of schizophrenia, called schizotypal personality disorder, tend to show special creative skills.[16]

---

[13] Huxley J et al. Schizophrenia as a genetic morphism. Nature 1964;204:220–1.

[14] Eduard, who his father called "Tete" (for petit), had a breakdown at about age 20 and was diagnosed with schizophrenia; he was eventually committed to an asylum. Robinson, Andrew (2015). Einstein: A Hundred Years of Relativity. Princeton University Press. pp. 143–145. ISBN 978-0-691-16989-7.

[15] Lucia Joyce was diagnosed with schizophrenia at the Burghölzli psychiatric clinic in Zurich.

[16] Fanous A, Kendler K. Genetic heterogeneity, modifier genes, and quantitative phenotypes in psychiatric illness: searching for a framework. Mol Psychiat 2005;10(1):6–13.

There is no question that genes play a very important role in the expression of schizophrenia. However, after considerable research those genes have not been identified. It is highly likely that there is a myriad of genes that contribute and the effect each gene has is varied and dependent on a number of factors. This would not support the balancing selection theory.

So we have the classification of a disorder called schizophrenia that is ill-defined and attempts to represent a spectrum of pathologic states genetically that are influenced to a varying and unknown extent by environmental factors. And from the evolutionary standpoint, it is unclear that it has existed long enough for evolutionary forces to influence its genetic transmission.

If this is the case for the most obvious of all mental disorder diagnoses, imagine the complexity to attempt an evolutionary explanation for all the other less well defined mental disorders that have much less genetic susceptibility than schizophrenia, some of which lead to death by suicide.

Although the genetic susceptibility for most mental disorders may be weak, there is without question genetic influence. Research into the genetics of psychiatric disorders indicates that while such alleles can predispose to developing a psychiatric condition under adverse environmental conditions such as childhood maltreatment, other variations can also protect, and in fact can allow enhanced coping upon encountering unfavorable environmental conditions during early stages of development[17].

---

[17] Brüne, M., Belsky, J., Fabrega, H., Feierman, J. R., Gilbert, P., Glantz, K., . . . Wilson, D. R. (2012). The crisis of psychiatry – insights and prospects from evolutionary theory. World Psychiatry, 11(1), 55-57.

For example, the "short" allele of the serotonin transporter coding gene is associated with greater risk for depression if linked with early childhood adversities, yet the same version of the gene is associated with reduced risk for depression if carriers grow up in emotionally secure conditions[18]. This suggests that evolution favored "plasticity" that renders individuals more susceptible to environmental contingencies – for better and worse[19]."

If evolution did not play a dominant role in the emergence of mental disorders, what did? In the next chapter we shall explore what has been written about mental disorders historically in order to arrive at some understanding of the time trajectory of its prevalence, epidemiology, and treatment.

This will bring into consideration the link of mental disorders with environmental factors, specifically dietary patterns.

---

[18] Belsky, J., & Pluess, M. (2009). Beyond diathesis stress: Differential susceptibility to environmental influences. Psychological Bulletin, 135(6), 885-908. doi:10.1037/a0017376.

[19] Belsky, J., Jonassaint, C., Pluess, M., Stanton, M., Brummett, B., & Williams, R. (2009). Vulnerability genes or plasticity genes? Molecular Psychiatry, 14(8), 746-754. doi:10.1038/mp.2009.44.

CHAPTER 2

Historical Perspective on Mood and Food

"Der Mensch ist was er isst."

(One is what one eats)

Ludwig Feuerbach

INTRODUCTION

If the emergence of mental disorders is relatively new in our evolution, just how new and how fast is it evolving? In this chapter we shall explore the prevalence of mental disorders throughout written history. As will be shown, it appears there has been a substantial increase in mental illness quite recently that is reaching crisis levels. Examination of this increase historically and geographically could lead to some clues as to how to reduce its prevalence.

The first healing intervention began when one man attempted to relieve another man's suffering by influencing him. This almost certainly predates written language, perhaps even language itself. There is healing from compassionate communication, a vanishing art in today's medicine.

TREPANATION

Trepanation is the practice of making a hole in the human skull exposing the brain's dura mater – the oldest known surgical procedure for which there is archeologic evidence. It is thought that perhaps these holes were drilled into a person who was behaving abnormally to let out what they believed were evil spirits.[20] Evidence of trepanation has been found in many prehistoric human remains from Neolithic times forward. Cave paintings seem to indicate that people believed the practice would cure seizures, migraines and mental disorders[21].

This could place the first evidence of mental illness about 10 thousand years ago.

EARLIEST HISTORICAL RECORDS OF MOOD DISORDER

The earliest known writings were perhaps the sixteen distinct markings known as Jiahu[22] symbols dating back to 6600 BC. There were a number of other symbolic markings, signs, and scripts that appear prior to a true writing system roughly corresponding to the emergence of the Bronze Age at about

---

[20] Nolen-Hoeksema (2014). *Abnormal psychology*, 6e. McGraw-Hill Education.

[21] Brothwell, Don R. (1963). *Digging up Bones; the Excavation, Treatment and Study of Human Skeletal Remains*. London: British Museum (Natural History). p. 126.

[22] Li, X; Harbottle, Garman; Zhang Juzhong; Wang Changsui (2003). "The earliest writing? Sign use in the seventh millennium BC at Jiahu, Henan Province, China". *Antiquity* 77 (295): 31–44.

3400 BC[23]. At that time, the first recorded histories began with that of the pharaohs and ancient Egypt.

The Ebers papyrus of 1550 BC, one of the most important medical papyri of ancient Egypt, mentions what appears to be clinical depression.[24]

The ancient Egyptian priest, Imhotep (c. 2650 – 2600 BC) was said to have used healing sanctuaries to heal people with physical and mental disorders, most of which today would be classified as psychological problems. These hospital-like structures were called "Dream Temples," and the effect they had upon participants has been likened to hypnosis; therefore, this may have been one of the first recorded formal psychological treatments.

In Homer's poems, written about 1000 BC, people suffering from mood disorders were thought to have offended the gods, who punished them by causing them to behave strangely[25]. Thus, when deranged, Ulysses plowed sand instead of fields and Ajax killed sheep instead of his enemies. Homer's Odyssey refers to an antidepressant potion, "*Nepenthes pharmakon,*" given to Helen of Troy by an Egyptian queen, Nepenthe, literally meaning "without grief" (*ne* = not, *penthos* = grief), pharmakon meaning remedy. This is likely a mythological drug that quells all sorrows with forgetfulness. Note the idea of a depressed mood state originating from thoughts of one's past.

---

[23] Smail, D. (2008) *On deep history and the brain.* An Ahmanson foundation book in the humanities. Berkeley: University of California Press.

[24] Scholl, Reinhold (2002). *Der Papyrus Ebers. Die größte Buchrolle zur Heilkunde Altägyptens.* Leipzig.

[25] Franz ,G. A. and Sheldon, T. Selesnick (1966). *The history of psychiatry: An evaluation of psychiatric thought and practice from prehistoric times to the present, p.27.* New York: Harper & Row.

AYURVEDA

In the Indian subcontinent, Ayurveda (life-knowledge) therapies have evolved over millennia[26]. These therapies employ specific plant foods for a variety of physical and mood states and is still used today.

The compendia of Caraka[27] constitute an important source of knowledge of Ayurveda. Insanity to Caraka was

> *"The unsettled condition of the mind, understanding, consciousness, perception, and memory."*

Etiologic factors included faulty diet, disrespect towards the gods, mental shock, and faulty bodily activities.

Therapeutic measures for insanity included medicinal herbs of colocynth, pepper, valerian, turmeric, cardamom, pomegranate, cinnamon leaf, sandalwood, garlic, jejube, radish, ginger, and asafetida[28]. *Rauvolfia serpentina*, or Indian snakeroot was a popular drug for insanity. A derivative of this compound (brand name Thorazine or generic chlorpromazine) revolutionized psychiatry in Western medicine and began the field of psychopharmocology.

---

[26] Meulenbeld, Gerrit Jan (1999). "Introduction". *A History of Indian Medical Literature*. Groningen: Egbert Forsten.

[27] Caraka, S. (1949). *Cikitsasthaba*, Vol 1 – 5, Jamnagar, India: Shree Guleb Kunverba Ayurvedic Society. Original at least from 6th century BC.

[28] Howells, J. G. (1975). World History of Psychiatry, p. 635, Brunner/ Mazel Publishers, New York.

Caraka writes

> *"The man of a strong mind who abstains from flesh and alcohol, observes a wholesome diet and is always dutiful and pure will never fall a victim to insanity."*

BIBLICAL

Malignant demons were considered the cause of mood disorders, asthma, and other more obscure conditions in Biblical accounts of ancient Judaic society. In the Talmud, however, supernatural powers have decreased emphasis, and the influence of the Talmud made Hebraic medicine less magical than was the medicine of ancient Babylon and Egypt. The Hebraic concern for the sick has always been an important influence on the humanitarian aspects of medicine and psychiatry, and as early as AD 490 there was a hospital in Jerusalem solely for the mentally ill[29]. In Deuteronomy 6:5 is written,

"The Lord will smite thee with madness,"

which indicates that although demons were considered the cause of insanity, the supreme controlling force was considered to be Divine.

Saul's mental illness, which is described in the first book of Samuel, was thought to have been caused by an evil spirit. Overcome with depression, Saul tried to persuade his servant to kill him; when the servant refused, Saul committed suicide (see 1 Samuel 31:4). There are also several biblical descriptions of catatonic excitement and epileptic fits[30].

---

[29] Alexander, F., & and Selesnick, S. T. (1966). *The history of psychiatry: an evaluation of psychiatric thought and practice from prehistoric times to the present* (p.23). New York: Harper & Row.

[30] Ibid.

Ezekiel 47:22 states

> *"Their fruit will be for food and their leaves for medicine."*

This appears in various ancient texts as the distinction between food for sustenance and medicinal properties and is associated with the sweetness/ bitterness ratio. Generally, the sweeter the plant, such as the fruit, the safer to eat and the higher the caloric density, preferred from an evolutionary standpoint. The more bitter the plant part, such as the leaves, the higher the likelihood of toxicity; however, remarkably for humans, the more likely the presence of healthful and restorative phytonutrients[31].

The Biblical Book of Daniel tells the tale of Daniel and a few friends who were visiting the king of Babylon who used meat that was ritualistically sacrificed in worship of the Babylonian gods. Daniel, not wishing to eat foods forbidden by God, requests only a plant based diet. In twenty-one days, it is noted that they are of good personal appearance and physical and mental health, compared to those who had indulged in the royal meaty foods.

HIPPOCRATES

Classical Greek thinking made possible the development of the natural sciences - the rationalistic approach in the "classical era". Cosmologic study shifted to the study of man around the

---

[31] All animals dislike bitter taste; carnivores will not eat bitter food. Certainly a wise meal balances the presence of bitter with sweet ala "a spoonful of sugar helps the medicine go down," song from Mary Poppins composed by Robert B. Sherman and Richard M. Sherman in 1964.

time of Hippocrates (460 - 370 BC), who considered by many to be the father of Western medicine.

Hippocrates separated the discipline of medicine from religion, arguing that disease was not a punishment inflicted by the gods but rather the product of environmental factors, diet, and lifestyle. The therapeutic approach was based on "the healing power of nature" (*vis medicatrix naturae*), that is, nature heals the patient with the physician as an assistant. According to this doctrine, the body contains within itself the power to rebalance and heal.

Hippocrates, allegedly stated:

> *"Let food be thy medicine and medicine thy food."*

This statement, having added meaning in today's Western world as will be detailed in this book, does not appear in any of the writings of Hippocrates including the *Hippocratic Corpus*[32], a heterogeneous compilation of sixty medical texts. In these texts, the definition between food and medicine (pharmaka) is unclear but, in any case, each was plant-derived. Medication often had a purgative effect, was quite bitter with a "strong" taste. There appears to be a correspondence to today's typical definition of "herb" (green leafy parts of plants with strong, often bitter taste) and spices (any other part of the plant other than leaves).

The *Hippocratic Corpus* does not have any book that is devoted entirely to pharmacology, although it does refer to "*Pharmakitides*", recipe books that have now been lost.

---

[32] Adams, Francis (1891). *The Genuine Works of Hippocrates*. New York: William Wood and Company.

For example, Hippocrates prescribed garlic for a variety of conditions including pulmonary complaints, as a cleansing agent, and for abdominal growths. Garlic was given to the original Olympic athletes in Greece as perhaps one of the earliest "performance enhancing" agents[33]. It is known today to influence a wide variety of ailments, including vascular disease, cancer, hepatic and microbial infections, to name but a few[34].

There was a strong continuum between dietetics and pharmacology in the ancient world.[35]

THE MEDIEVAL PERIOD

Years of internal wars amongst the Greek city-states which differed politically weakened Greece. After Alexander the Great, the Romans rose to power and defeated Greece. The Romans adopted the intellectual heritage of Greece but focused on technical and military might. Then came epidemics. Between the first and fourth centuries AD three epidemics each killed much of Western civilization. The deadly chaos of the time was comforted by Christianity. Christian priests gave advice on healing diseases as well as saving souls. In the fourth century AD an alliance between church and state was

---

[33] Green, O., & Polydoris, N. (1993). *Garlic, cancer and heart disease: Review and recommendations*, pp. 21-41. Chicago, Ill.: GN Communications (Pub.).

[34] Banerjee, S., Mukherjee, P., & Maulik, S. (2003). Garlic as an antioxidant: The good, the bad and the ugly. *Phytotherapy Research Phytother. Res., 17*(2), 97-106.

[35] Totelin, L. (2015). When foods become remedies in ancient Greece: The curious case of garlic and other substances. *Journal of Ethnopharmacology, 167*, 30-37. doi:10.1016/j.jep.2014.08.018.

established as Charlemagne was christened emperor of the Holy Roman Empire.

The positive consoling influence of the Church gave renewed conviction to the demoralized citizenry. However, there was a distinct clash of the scientific, the rational, with the mysticism of faith. Mental health recognition regressed to prescientific demonology and its treatment to forms of exorcism.

So it was for more than a millennium – until the Renaissance.

THE RENAISSANCE

In the fourteenth and early fifteenth centuries plagues, famines, wars, and corrupt clergical practices influenced a reemergence of classical thought but with a twist: the recognition of the value of one's own thinking/ creativity. This was fueled by the printing press, the discovery of new continents, new trade routes and prosperity.

Unfortunately, the world of mental health remained in the mystical realm, although in the latter years of this period did shift toward alchemy in which substances – salts, sulfur, and mercury – were prescribed in simple exact dosages for certain emotional conditions. Although those concoctions were not in themselves helpful, the approach to the person as an individual was established during the Renaissance - the vital principle of objective observation of the patient as an individual.

THE ENLIGHTENMENT

The eighteenth century saw a blossoming of scientific experimentation rather than philosophic thought. It was appreciated that there are no "laws" of nature, only mathematical representations of experimental facts. Classification and description of diseases became highly useful to diagnose and then treat based on the diagnosis and successful experiments with those diseases. The exceptions were mental disorders, being too varied and complex in presentation to neatly classify and with no identifiable "lesion." This remains largely true even today although a classification system has regularly expanded to create – artificially – more and more classification[36].

To at least the year 1700, cases of "insanity" seldom included reported auditory hallucinations. Psychosis was relatively brief, affected patients of any age, and often occurred in the presence of other diseases[37]. The prevailing descriptions of emotional turmoil appear to be melancholia or mild to moderate clinical depression. Suicide was either rare or rarely described.

THE MODERN ERA

In the eighteenth century, there was no organized way to treat mental illness – or the demented and cognitively compromised. Families of the affected were expected to manage these individuals as best they could. Unfortunately, those severely affected were so burdensome that there was often abusive treatment including abandonment. Those abandoned in this way would wander through the countryside and be scorned, ridiculed and beaten.

The asylums of the late eighteenth and nineteenth century did provide a partial solution, at least from the standpoint of placement. However, there was abuse there too. Here is a typical description of the setting:

---

[36] DSM series.

[37] Torrey, E. F., & Miller, J. (2001). The invisible plague: the rise of mental illness from 1750 to the present. New Jersey: Rutgers University Press.

"strong chains were employed to hold the excited patients. These chains, fixed at different heights to the sides of stoves, have iron rings at the end, by means of which the arms or the legs of the patient are rendered completely immovable. Far from fearing that a painful impression will be produced on the patients by chains, they think, on the contrary, that this apparatus exerts a beneficial influence upon them; that it intimidates, humbles them, and removes all desire to attempt to get rid of their fastenings.[38]"

Not only mechanical restraint, but primitive "treatment" consisted of administering substances or procedures that would cause loss of blood, emesis or diarrhea, with the thought that evacuation would carry the disease from the body. For example, mercury was offered for this purpose; of course later it was discovered, ironically, that mercury poisoning *causes* psychosis. The phrase "mad as a hatter", from the millinery trade, utilized mercury in the processing of the felt in the manufacture of hats, leading to psychosis in some workers.

A major advancement in the treatment of such institutionalized patients began with the so-called "moral treatment" of Philippe Pinel[39] and William Tuke[40], exemplified in the following account:

---

[38] Tuke, D. H. (1882) Chapters in the history of the insane in the British Isles, p.140. Kegan Paul Trench and Company, London.

[39] Pinel, Philippe (1806). A treatise on insanity: In which are contained the principles of a new and more practical nosology of maniacal disorders than has yet been offered to the public. Sheffield, England: W. Todd.

"He was calm; his attention appeared to be arrested by his new situation ... the superintendent conducted him to his (room), and told him the circumstances on which his treatment would depend; that it was his wish to make every inhabitant in the house as comfortable as possible and that he sincerely hoped the patient's conduct would render it unnecessary for him to have recourse to coercion. The (patient) was sensible of the kindness of his treatment. He promised to restrain himself, and he so completely succeeded, that, during his stay, no coercive means were ever employed towards him. ... The superintendent on these occasions went to his (room); and though the first sight of him seemed rather to increase the patient's irritation, yet after sitting some time quietly beside him, the violent excitement subsided, and he would listen with attention to the persuasions and arguments of his friendly visitor. After such conversations, the patient was generally better for some days or a week; and in about four months he was discharged perfectly recovered."[41]

---

[40] Tuke, Samuel [1813] (1996). Description of the Retreat. London: Process Press.

[41] Tuke, S. (1813), *The Retreat, an institution near York for insane persons*(p. 147). W. Alexander Publis.

In the United States, the beginnings of institutionalized care of the mentally ill had beginnings at the New York Hospital founded in 1771 with a charter from King George III; construction was slowed by the American Revolutionary War. In 1798, the governors announced that the Hospital was primarily for the purpose of medical treatment, secondly for surgical treatment and thirdly for treatment of "maniacs[42]." Accounts indicate that there were only a couple of dozen patients considered to have psychiatric issues and these were moved from the New York Hospital to the Bloomindale Insane Asylum in 1821; the Asylum was increased in size by 30 beds in 1829 and another 30 beds in 1837[43]. That is a total of about 80 beds in one of the first and largest mental hospitals in the United States.

The Madness of King George

King George III not only subsidized the first "insane asylums" in the United States, he himself apparently became "mad" – some accounts state that the condition was porphyria, a disease of the blood treated by, among other things, a high carbohydrate diet and blood-letting. This is one of the very few examples of an aberrant mental condition for which blood-letting, a common treatment at the time for all mental disorders, might actually have led to improvement.

---

[42] Stone, W. L. (1872). *History of New York City from the discovery to the present day (p.231)*. Virtue and Yorston, New York.

[43] Earle, P. (1843). *History, description, and statistics of the Bloomingdale Asylum for the Insane (p. 12)*. Egbert, Hovey and King, Printers, New York.

It has been proposed that before approximately 1750, mental disorders severe enough to require hospitalization were caused by many medical conditions (for example, brain tumors, alcoholic encephalitis, stroke, dementia) and that it had a stable baseline rate of about 1 person per 1000[44]. The prevalence of mental disorders began to exceed this baseline in the middle of the nineteenth century and continued to rise unabated for 100 years.

In 1808, Professor Dr. Johann Christian Reil, a German physician, was first to use the term "psychiatry" (in German, *psychiaterie*)˙ and suggested that there be a distinct field of medicine devoted to the mentally ill.

RECENT HISTORY OF MOOD DISORDER PREVALENCE

Some idea of this increase might be illustrated by the accompanying Figure 1. In that figure, the number of hospitalized patients is plotted versus the year from 1850 to 1954[45]. Generally, it can be appreciated that the numbers significantly increased with time, approximately by a factor of three over that hundred-year span.

---

[44] Torrey, E.F. & Miller, J. (2001). *The invisible plague: the rise of mental illness from 1750 to the present.* New Brunswick, NJ: Rutgers University Press.

[45] "Timeline: Treatments for Mental Illness." (n.d.). American Experience, History television series PBS . Accessed June, 2016.

Figure 1 Mentally Ill Hospitalized Patients

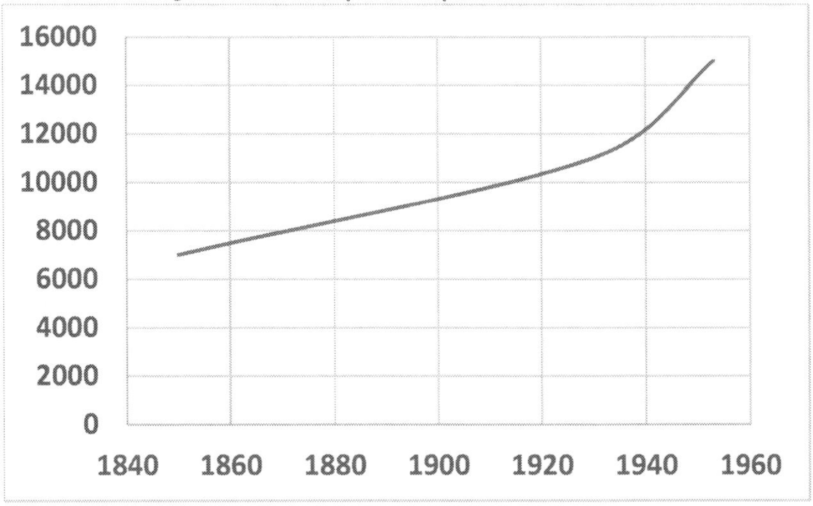

A number of factors could be confounding these data, however. For example, the causes of many admissions in the nineteenth century were actually for medical reasons; "general paresis of the insane" being one of the most common diagnoses, later understood to be caused by neurosyphillus. On the other hand, the increasing availability of facilities may have allowed an expansion of the patients admitted, although it could be argued that expansion was driven by demand.

More recent data from the National Health Survey in 1989 indicate a prevalence of severe mental illness of 18.2 per 1000 population[46]. Although definitions of what constitutes severe mental illness – or the application of criteria - may have varied from the middle of the nineteenth century, an 18-fold increase is significant. Figure 2, titled "Severe Mental Illness" illustrates

---

[46] Barker PR, Manderscheid RW, Hendershot GE, Jack SS, Schoenborn CA, Goldstrom I; Division of Health Interview Statistics, National Center for Health Statistics. Serious mental illness and disability in the adult household population: United States, 1989. Adv Data 1992;(218):1–11.

this trend from 1750 to 1989; an exponential increase in prevalence is apparent.

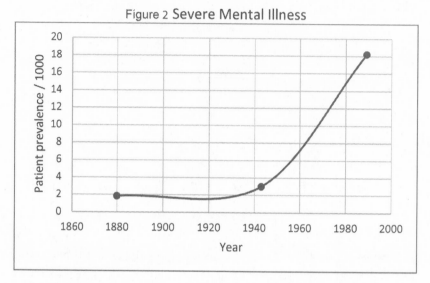

Figure 2 Severe Mental Illness

The National Comorbidity Survey[47] (United States) conducted in 1990 - 1992 was the first survey using a structured psychiatric interview in a national sample. This survey indicated a mood disorder prevalence of 113 per 1000 individuals. A study of over 10,000 Taiwanese[48] had a prevalence of only 9.

[47] Kessler, R. C. (1994). Lifetime and 12-Month Prevalence of DSM-III-R Psychiatric Disorders in the United States. Archives of General Psychiatry, 51(1), 8. doi:10.1001/archpsyc.1994.03950010008002

[48] Hwu, H., Yeh, E., & Chang, L. (1989). Prevalence of psychiatric disorders in Taiwan defined by the Chinese Diagnostic Interview Schedule. Acta Psychiatrica Scandinavica Acta Psychiatr Scand, 79(2), 136-147. doi:10.1111/j.1600-0447.1989.tb08581.x

The WHO World Mental Health Survey Consortium conducted face-to-face interviews of 60,463 adults during 2001 – 2003 in 14 countries around the world[49] using DSM-IV criteria[50]. Some of the results are shown in the accompany table where

Figure 3 Mood Disorder per 1000

Country	mood
US	96
France	85
Italy	38
Spain	49
Japan	31
Nigeria	8
China	25

prevalence of mood disorders (figures are again numbers per 1000 surveyed individuals) for a sample of the countries surveyed. Western "developed" countries such as the United States and France had a relatively high incidence of mood disorders, while the Mediterranean countries of Spain and Italy significantly lower prevalence. Japan and China was seen to have even lower prevalence, while "underdeveloped" countries such as Nigeria had the lowest prevalence.

---

[49] The WHO World Mental Health Survey Consortium. Prevalence, Severity, and Unmet Need for Treatment of Mental Disorders in the World Health Organization World Mental Health Surveys. *JAMA.* 2004;291(21):2581-2590. doi:10.1001/jama.291.21.258.

[50] American Psychiatric Association. (2000). *Diagnostic and statistical manual of mental disorders* (4th ed., text rev.). Washington, DC.

An epidemiologic survey of psychiatric disorders in Iran[51] reported a prevalence of 11%. While that survey was performed using somewhat different criteria than the above studies, it is an important representation of a non-Western Middle Eastern country with much different epidemiologic variables and an apparent relatively low prevalence of psychiatric disorders.

Many studies have found that recent generations are more likely to meet the criteria for mood disorders. For example, in the United States, one study showed 1–2% of people born early in the 20th century reporting clinical depression, compared to more than 15–20% of those born after the middle of the century[52]. Between 1987 and 1997, the percentage of Americans in whom depression was diagnosed and treated more than tripled[53].

The primary cause of disability in the United States and the rest of the world is depression[54]. The World Health Organization

---

[51] Mohammadi MR, Davidian H, Noorbala AA et al. (2005) An epide-miological survey of psychiatric disorders in Iran. Clin Pract Epidemiol Ment Health 1, 16.

[52] Twenge, J. M., Gentile, B., DeWall, C. N., Ma, D., Lacefield, K., & Schurtz, D. R. (2010). Birth cohort increases in psychopathology among young Americans, 1938–2007: A cross-temporal meta-analysis of the MMPI. *Clinical Psychology Review, 30*(2), 145-154. doi:10.1016/j.cpr.2009.10.005.

[53] Olfson, M. (2002). National Trends in the Outpatient Treatment of Depression. Jama, 287(2), 203. doi:10.1001/jama.287.2.203.

[54] Murray CJL, Lopez AD, eds. (1996). The global burden of disease: a comprehensive assessment of mortality and disability from disease, inju-ries and risk factors in 1990 and projected to 2020. Global Burden of Disease and Injury Series. Vol 1. Cambridge, Mass: Harvard University Press.

predicts that by 2020, depression will be second only to heart disease as a cause of premature death and disability[55].

Therefore, it is apparent that the prevalence of mood disorders is increasing rapidly. Among Westernized societies, the Mediterranean countries and Japan have the lowest prevalence. Non Westernized relatively "undeveloped" counties such as Taiwan and Nigeria have the lowest prevalence.

MOOD AND FOOD

Why is the prevalence of psychiatric disorders increasing so rapidly and why is it that the prevalence is so much greater in the Westernized countries compared to those countries with more traditional diets?

Western diets are linked to higher consumption of energy-dense, nutrient-poor foods and beverages. The highly palatable combination of sugar, fat and salt plays a key role in the attractiveness of such foods[56] [57]. The traditional diets of the Mediterranean countires, Japanese, Taiwanese and the Chinese may have survived the initial influences of Westernization

---

[55] The burden of disease: Global burden of disease and injury attributable to selected risk factors, 1990. (2002). Bmj, 325(7370), 928-928. doi:10.1136/bmj.325.7370.928.

[56] . Lindberg MA, Dementieva Y, Cavender J: Why has the BMI gone up so drastically in the last 35 years? J Addict Med 2011, 5:272–278.

[57] Morgan, D., & Sizemore, G. M. (2011). Animal Models of Addiction: Fat and Sugar. CPD Current Pharmaceutical Design, 17(12), 1168-1172. doi:10.2174/138161211795656747.

because of cultural traditions. The diets of developing countries also remain more traditional.

Is there an influence that dietary patterns might have on mood states. Is so, why? An attempt at explaining this possible correlation requires that we probe into basic physiologic mechanisms; we shall do this is the next few chapters – while indicating specific suggestions of the protective and healing power of plants.

Part II WHY

Why are psychiatric disturbances increasing at such a rapid rate in our society? What are the root causes of cognitive and emotional problems and what can be done to prevent, alleviate, and eliminate these problems?

CHAPTER 3

Nutritional Programming and Mood throughout the Lifespan

"You may be an undigested bit of beef, a blot of mustard, a crumb of cheese, a fragment of underdone potato. There's more of gravy than of grave about you, whatever you are!"

Charles Dickens, *A Christmas Carol*

INTRODUCTION

In the last chapter three facts were discovered:

- Psychiatric disorders, such as adverse mood states, are a relatively recent phenomenon in our evolution.

- The prevalence of these disorders appears to be accelerating.
- Countries with more traditional diets have lower mental disorder prevalence than Westernized countries.

In this chapter we shall more closely examine the nutritional epidemiology of dietary patterns on mood states. Studies of single nutrients on mood states are trickier as they do not consider the complex interactions between nutrients. That we shall review in Part III.

ADULT DIETARY PATTERNS AND MOOD

Even though most medications used in psychiatry are derived directly from plant secondary metabolites or patented variations, only very recently have psychiatrists begun to consider the healing power of plants themselves. The March 2010 issue of the so-called "green journal," a most prestigious and conservative journal of the American Psychiatric Association actually featured dietary considerations as related to psychiatric disorders.

An editorial appeared in that issue written by Marlene Freeman, MD and Associate Professor in the Department of Psychiatry at Harvard Medical School, in which she notes:

> *"It is both compelling and daunting that dietary interventions at an individual or population level could reduce rates of psychiatric disorders."*

One such study in that issue is titled "Association of Western and Traditional Diets with Depression and Anxiety in Women[58]." In this and all research into the relationship

---

[58] Jacka, F. N., Pasco, J. a, Mykletun, A., Williams, L. J., Hodge, A. M., O'Reilly, S. L., ... Berk, M. (2010). Association of Western and traditional

between diet quality and emotional states, there is always the challenge of *defining* and *measuring* diet quality and mood. There is no accepted "gold standard" measure of either.

With that in mind, this was a study of about one thousand adult women who were examined over a short time interval, a so-called cross-sectional study. Their conclusion was that:

> *"a 'traditional' dietary pattern characterized by vegetables, fruit, meat, fish, and whole grains was associated with lower odds for major de-pression or dysthymia and for anxiety disorders. A "Western" diet of processed or fried foods, re-fined grains, sugary products, and beer was as-sociated with a higher GHQ-12 score."*

The GHQ-12 is just one of those measures of emotional health, a 12-item questionnaire asked of each subject participant – the lower the score the better. More generally, the authors state:

> *"There was also an inverse association between diet quality score and GHQ-12 score."*

Again "diet quality" was defined by a particular food frequency questionnaire utilized, so by their definitions, a better diet quality resulted in better emotional states. By their measures, a "Western Diet" is of low diet quality and a "Traditional Diet" is of higher diet quality.

Another study looking at the relationship of diet to mood in adults is titled "Dietary pattern and depressive symptoms in

---

diets with depression and anxiety in women. The American Journal of Psychiatry, 167(3), 305–11.

middle age[59]." This work followed more than three thousand participants over a five-year time interval whose dietary habits fell into one of two categories:

> " 'whole food' (heavily loaded by vegetables, fruits and fish) and 'processed food' (heavily loaded by sweetened desserts, fried food, processed meat, refined grains and high-fat dairy products)."

At the end of the five years, depressive symptomatology was measured by a selected instrument called "CES-D". Their conclusion was that:

> "In middle-aged participants, a processed food dietary pattern is a risk factor for CES–D depression 5 years later, whereas a whole food pattern is protective."

On the other hand, when the "processed food dietary pattern" is followed extensively, the odds of becoming depressed are significantly increased, a risk factor for depression. Within the limitations of the study, these results are statistically significant and rather dramatic.

Another large prospective cohort study performed at the University College London[60] showed a significant correlation

---

[59] Akbaraly, T. N., Brunner, E. J., Ferrie, J. E., Marmot, M. G., Kivimaki, M., & Singh-Manoux, A. (2009). Dietary pattern and depressive symptoms in middle age. The British Journal of Psychiatry : The Journal of Mental Science, 195(5), 408–13. doi:10.1192/bjp.bp.108.058925.

[60] Akbaraly, T. N., Sabia, S., Shipley, M. J., Batty, G. D., & Kivimaki, M. (2013). Adherence to healthy dietary guidelines and future depressive symptoms: evidence for sex differentials in the Whitehall II study. The American Journal of Clinical Nutrition, 97(2), 419–27.

between a healthy diet and the lack of depressive symptoms in women over a five-year time interval.

A "healthy diet" was based on the Harvard Alternative Healthy Eating Index which emphasizes vegetables and fruits, low fat and oils, protein from sources such as fish, nuts, and seeds; it does, however, allow for inclusion of meat and dairy but less so than the current USDA recommendations. Depressive symptoms were based on the Center for Epidemiologic Studies Depression Scale.

Their conclusion was that

> *"There was a suggestion that a poor diet is a risk factor for future depression in women."*

There was a positive dose-response nature as well, i.e., the healthier the diet the less the odds of developing sustained depressive symptoms over the five-year interval.

There are a number of other studies that make similar claims of improving mood in adults with better dietary patterns, such as a study performed at the University of Delaware reported in 2010[61], which concludes

> *"Diet quality was significantly associated with reported symptoms of depression."*

---

[61] Kuczmarski, M. F., Cremer Sees, A., Hotchkiss, L., Cotugna, N., Evans, M. K., & Zonderman, A. B. (2010). Higher Healthy Eating Index-2005 scores associated with reduced symptoms of depression in an urban population: findings from the Healthy Aging in Neighborhoods of Diversity Across the Life Span (HANDLS) study. Journal of the American Dietetic Association, 110(3), 383–9.

And another at the University of Calgary in 2012[62] stating their study

> *"was consistent with prior epidemiologic surveys, revealing an association between higher levels of nutrient intakes and better mental health."*

There is an association between dietary patterns, diabetes, and depression[63]. Type 2 diabetes and depression are commonly comorbid high-prevalence chronic disorders. Diet is a key diabetes risk factor and research has highlighted the relevance of diet as a possible risk factor for common mental disorders. A Healthy Diet, characterized by vegetables, leafy greens, fruit, cooked whole grains, and whole grain bread, was found to be a protective factor, while an Unhealthy Diet, characterized by the consumption of fried potatoes, cheese, red meat, processed meats, pizza, non-fried potatoes, and regular soft drinks was associated with increased risk for depression in those with or without type 2 diabetes.

THE MEDITERRANEAN DIET

One particularly well-studied dietary pattern considered by some as a "healthy diet" is the *Mediterranean Diet*. This diet was inspired by the traditional dietary patterns of Greece, Spain and Southern Italy. These countries are the biggest olive producing countries, so it is no wonder that the diet features olive oil.

---

[62] Davison, K. M., & Kaplan, B. J. (2012). Nutrient intakes are correlated with overall psychiatric functioning in adults with mood disorders. Canadian Journal of Psychiatry. Revue Canadienne de Psychiatrie, 57(2), 85–92.

[63] Dipnall, J. F., Pasco, J. A., Meyer, D., Berk, M., Williams, L. J., Dodd, S., & Jacka, F. N. (2015). The association between dietary patterns, diabetes and depression. *Journal Of Affective Disorders, 174215-224.* doi:10.1016/j.jad.2014.11.030.

The principal aspects of this diet include proportionally high consumption of olive oil, legumes, unrefined cereals, fruits and vegetables, moderate to high consumption of fish, moderate consumption of dairy products, moderate wine consumption, and low consumption of meat and animal products.

This particular diet has been chosen for a number of psychiatric studies because the lifetime prevalence of mental disorders has been found to be lower in Mediterranean countries than in Northern European countries. Suicide rates, which may indirectly reflect the prevalence of severe depression, tend also to be lowest in Mediterranean countries.

One such study of the Mediterranean Diet, published in 2009 by a group at a Spanish University[64] examined over 10,000 participants using physicians' clinical diagnoses of mood disorder and the extent of adherence to the Mediterranean Diet over an average time interval of more than four years. A self-reported physician-provided diagnosis of depression demonstrated acceptable validity using the Structured Clinical Interview for the Diagnostic and Statistical Manual of Mental Disorders fourth edition by experienced psychiatrists blinded to the answers to the questionnaires. They concluded that their results

> *"suggest a potential protective role of the Mediterranean Diet with regard to the prevention of depressive disorders."*

These same researchers extended their prospective study out

---

[64] Sánchez-Villegas, A., Delgado-Rodríguez, M., Alonso, A., Schlatter, J., Lahortiga, F., Serra Majem, L., & Martínez-González, M. A. (2009). Association of the Mediterranean dietary pattern with the incidence of depression: the Seguimiento Universidad de Navarra/University of Navarra follow-up (SUN) cohort. Archives of General Psychiatry, 66(10), 1090–8.

to ten years[65]. They examined again the Mediterranean Diet but also a "Pro-vegetarian Dietary Pattern" which basically is a non-strict vegetarian diet. Both of these dietary patterns proved protective from mood disorders, with the Pro-vegetarian Diet superior to the Mediterranean Diet. Interestingly, there was a "dose response" effect in that low adherence to these diets had much less of an effect than a moderate adherence.

Another large prospective cohort epidemiologic investigation was reported recently from researchers at Loma Linda University[66]. Their conclusion was that

> *"foods typical of Mediterranean diets were associated with positive affect as well as lower negative affect while Western foods were associated with low positive affect in general and negative affect in women."*

Scientists in Iran compared prevalence of depression in Iranians with a traditional Iranian diet versus the emerging Western dietary pattern[67]. They used a validated semi-quantitative food frequency questionnaire and a Hospital Anxiety and Depression

---

[65] Sánchez-Villegas, A., Henríquez-Sánchez, P., Ruiz-Canela, M., La-hortiga, F., Molero, P., Toledo, E., & Martínez-González, M. A. (2015). A longitudinal analysis of diet quality scores and the risk of incident depression in the SUN Project. *BMC Medicine, 13*(1), 1-12. doi:10.1186/s12916-015-0428-y.

[66] Ford, P. A., Jaceldo-Siegl, K., Lee, J. W., Youngberg, W., & Tonstad, S. (2013). Intake of Mediterranean foods associated with positive affect and low negative affect. Journal of Psychosomatic Research, 74(2), 142–8.

[67] Hosseinzadeh, M., Vafa, M., Esmaillzadeh, A., Feizi, A., Majdzadeh, R., Afshar, H., & ... Adibi, P. (2016). Empirically derived dietary patterns in relation to psychological disorders. *Public Health Nutrition, 19*(2), 204-217. doi:10.1017/S136898001500172X.

Scale. Their conclusion was to reduce the influence of the Western dietary pattern:

> *"Recommendation to increase the intake of fruits, citrus fruits, vegetables, and low-fat dairy products and to reduce the intakes of snacks, high-fat dairy products, chocolate, carbonated drinks, sweets and desserts might be associated with lower chance of psychological disorders."*

Even short term adherence to a Mediterranean-style diet may benefit psychological functioning. One study assessed the impact of switching to a ten-day Mediterranean-style diet on mood and cognition[68]. Utilizing a crossover design, in which subjects first have or do not have the Mediterranean Diet for ten days, then switch to the other diet for ten days, the Mediterranean Diet was associated with significantly elevated contentment and alertness.

All the studies shown so far in the context of exploring mood states define dietary patterns in various ways but allow various amounts of most all foods. What about more restrictive diets such as vegetarian or even vegan? Very few studies exist.

VEGETARIAN DIET

Bonnie Beezhold and colleagues at Arizona State University conducted such a study but the motivation for it was the thought that vegetarian diets might be bad for brain function

---

[68] Lee, J., Pase, M., Pipingas, A., Raubenheimer, J., Thurgood, M., Villalon, L., & ... Scholey, A. (2015). Applied nutritional investigation. Switching to a 10-day Mediterranean-style diet improves mood and cardiovascular function in a controlled crossover study. *Nutrition*, *31*(5), 647-352. doi:10.1016/j.nut.2014.10.008

and mood states because they exclude fish, the major dietary source of *eicosapentaenoic acid* and *docosahexaenoic acid*, critical regulators of brain cell structure and function[69].

The investigators used a food frequency questionnaire and a psychometric test called the "Depression Anxiety Stress Scale" in a cross-sectional study.

Their conclusion was that

> *"The vegetarian diet profile does not appear to adversely affect mood despite low intake of long-chain omega-3 fatty acids."*

But the conclusion doesn't tell their whole story. Not only does the vegetarian diet not compromise mood states, results indicate a considerable advantage over an omnivore diet for female and males.

The same researches more recently reported a similar study but in this one, patients were randomly selected to receive three different diets over a two-week time interval[70]: typical omnivore, omnivore with only fish as the flesh food, and vegetarian.

Their conclusion was :

---

[69] Beezhold, B. L., Johnston, C. S., & Daigle, D. R. (2010). Vegetarian diets are associated with healthy mood states: a cross-sectional study in seventh day adventist adults. Nutrition Journal, 9, 26. doi:10.1186/1475-2891-9-26.

[70] Beezhold, B. L., & Johnston, C. S. (2012). Restriction of meat, fish, and poultry in omnivores improves mood: a pilot randomized controlled trial. *Nutrition Journal, 11*, 9. doi:10.1186/1475-2891-11-9.

> *"Restricting meat, fish, and poultry improved some domains of short-term mood state in modern omnivores. "*

And they are correct to point out the remarkable fact that

> *"this is the first trial to examine the impact of restricting meat, fish, and poultry on mood state in omnivores."*

A study performed in Puerto Rico compared a vegetarian population to a non-vegetarian population using three different scales for mood states.[71] Their conclusion was

> *"more anxiety and depression were reported in the non-vegetarian groups in comparison to the vegetarian group."*

The Beezhold studies also yielded some additional interesting results of the effect on anxiety. The randomly selected individuals who ate the vegetarian diet happened to score the highest in anxiety level at the beginning of the study but scored the lowest compared to those on the other diets after two weeks.

The same was true with a measure of fatigue; the group with the vegetarian diet was worst at the beginning and best at the end of the study.

---

[71] Rodríguez Jiménez, J., Rodríguez, J. R., & Gonzaléz, M. J. (1998). [Indicators of anxiety and depression in subjects with different kinds of diet: vegetarians and omnivores]. *Boletín De La Asociación Médica De Puerto Rico, 90*(4-6), 58-68.

VEGAN

An 18-week randomized controlled trial of adopting a low-fat vegan diet was performed at 10 GEICO corporate sites[72]. Mood states were measured using a 36-item Short Form Health Survey; this instrument is reliable and valid[73]. That study showed a statistically significant improvement in indicators for depression, anxiety, fatigue, and work productivity in those switching to the vegan diet for 18 weeks.

A survey of North American omnivores, vegetarians, and vegans using the Depression Anxiety Stress Scales – 21 revealed[74]:

> *"increasing restriction of animal foods (e.g. going from vegetarian to vegan) is associated with improved mood."*

ADOLESCENT DIETARY PATTERNS – JUNK FOOD, JUNK MOODS

Mental health issues are particularly important for adolescents, as the vulnerability to mental illness increases during times of transition from childhood to adolescence and then to

---

[72] Agarwal, U., Mishra, S., Jia, X., Levin, S., Gonzales, J., & Barnard, N. D. (2015). A Multicenter Randomized Controlled Trial of a Nutrition Intervention Program in a Multiethnic Adult Population in the Corporate Setting Reduces Depression and Anxiety and Improves Quality of Life: The GEICO Study. *American Journal Of Health Promotion, 29*(4), 245-254. doi:10.4278/ajhp.130218-QUAN-72.

[73] Ware, J. E. (2000). SF-36 Health Survey Update. Spine, 25(24), 3130-3139. doi:10.1097/00007632-200012150-00008

[74] Beezhold, B., Radnitz, C., Rinne, A., & DiMatteo, J. (2015). Vegans report less stress and anxiety than omnivores. *Nutritional Neuroscience, 18*(7), 289-296. doi:10.1179/1476830514Y.0000000164.

adulthood[75]. Around 50% of all lifetime mental disorders start by the age of 14[76].

Teen consumption of "junk foods" and other unhealthy dietary choices may be contributing significantly to the burgeoning mental health crisis in that age group.

Significant increases in the prevalence of adolescent emotional distress and behavioral problems have occurred over the past several generations.[77]

Paralleling this mental health pathology among young people is a reduction in the quality of adolescents' diets over recent generations with decreasing consumption of raw fruits, high-nutrient vegetables and associated increases in fast food, snacks and sweetened beverages[78] with resulting obesity[79].

While data are relatively scarce from randomized, controlled trials to demonstrate the efficacy of healthful eating on psychiatric disorders in adolescents, there is emerging epidemiologic evidence. Most of the literature based on

---

[75] Andersen, S. L. (2003). Trajectories of brain development: Point of vulnerability or window of opportunity? Neuroscience & Biobehavioral Reviews, 27(1-2), 3-18. doi:10.1016/s0149-7634(03)00005-8.

[76] Kessler, R. C., Berglund, P., Demler, O., Jin, R., Merikangas, K. R., & Walters, E. E. (2005). Lifetime Prevalence and Age-of-Onset Distributions of DSM-IV Disorders in the National Comorbidity Survey Replication. Archives of General Psychiatry, 62(6), 593. doi:10.1001/archpsyc.62.6.593.

[77] Twenge JM, Gentile B, DeWall CN, Lacefield K, et al. (2010) Birth cohort increases in psychopathology among young Americans, 1938–2007: A cross-temporal meta-analysis of the MMPI.Clin Psychol Rev 30: 145–154. 21.

[78] Cavadini C, Siega-Riz AM, Popkin BM (2000) US adolescent food intake trends from 1965 to 1996. West J Med 173: 378–383.

[79] Ogden CL, Flegal KM, Carroll MD, Johnson CL (2002) Prevalence and trends in overweight among US children and adolescents, 1999–2000. Jama 288: 1728–1732.

studies of adults appears to suggest similar correlations with adolescent diets.

Cross-sectional studies on the effect of diet quality on adolescents indicate an association between dietary patterns and mental health. Poorer emotional states and behavior were seen in adolescents with a typical Western dietary pattern high in red and processed meats, takeaway foods, confectionery and refined foods compared to those who consumed more fresh fruit and vegetables[80][81].

The first prospective cohort study on the effect of diet quality on mental health of adolescents was published in 2011, based on over 3000 adolescents ages 11- 18 years old[82]. Participants with poor diet quality at baseline had more emotional and behavioral problems; these worsened with time passage if a poor diet continued but improved if their diets improved. Those with good baseline diet quality had fewer psychiatric problems but if that diet deteriorated, so did their mental health. A healthy diet was defined as one that included fruit and vegetables as "core food groups" and included both two or more servings of fruit per day and four or more servings of vegetables, as well as general avoidance of junk food such as processed foods including chips, fried foods, chocolate, sweets, and ice cream.

---

[80] Oddy WH, Robinson M, Ambrosini GL, de Klerk NH, et al. (2009) The association between dietary patterns and mental health in early adolescence. Prev Med 49: 39–44.

[81] Jacka FN, Kremer PJ, Leslie E, Berk M, Patton G, et al. (2010) Associations between diet quality and depressed mood in adolescents: results from the Healthy Neighbourhoods study. Aust N Z J Psychiatry 44: 435–442. 10.

[82] Jacka FN, Kremer PJ, Berk M, de Silva-Sanigorski AM, Moodie M, et al. (2011) A prospective study of diet quality and mental health in adolescents. PLoS ONE 6(9).

In another prospective investigation, data were collected at two points in time (2001 and 2003) from nearly 3,000 adolescents, aged 11–12 years or 13–14 years, a group of ethnically diverse and socially deprived adolescents from East London in the United Kingdom[83]. Diet quality was measured from dietary questionnaires, and mental health assessed using the Strengths and Difficulties Questionnaire and the Short Mood and Feelings Questionnaire. Again, a healthy diet devoid of processed foods and rich in fruits and vegetables was associated with improved mood states.

A study of the association between dietary pattern and depression in adolescent females was performed using a Korean version of the Beck Depression Inventory (K-BDI) and the Food Frequency Questionnaire published by the Korean Health and Nutrition Examination Survey[84]. They found that:

> *"consumption of instant foods including ramen, hamburger, pizza, fried foods, and processed foods such as ham, fish paste, and snacks was associated with increased depression and was positively correlated to K-BDI scores in adolescent girls after adjusting for menstrual regularity and energy intake. By contrast, consumption of green vegetables and 1 to 3 servings/day of fruits was associated with decreased risk of depression."*

---

[83] Jacka, F., Rothon, C., Taylor, S., Berk, M., & Stansfeld, S. (2013). Diet quality and mental health problems in adolescents from East London: a prospective study. *Social Psychiatry & Psychiatric Epidemiology*, *48*(8), 1297-1306. doi:10.1007/s00127-012-0623-5.

[84] Kim, T., Choi, J., Lee, H., & Park, Y. (2015). Associations between Dietary Pattern and Depression in Korean Adolescent Girls. *Journal Of Pediatric & Adolescent Gynecology*, *28*(6), 533-537. doi:10.1016/j.jpag.2015.04.005.

Another study was performed in the People's Republic of China to determine the association between major dietary patterns and the risk of depression in Chinese adolescents[85]. Three major dietary patterns were identified in the study based on factor analysis which they termed "snack", "animal food", and "traditional." Results indicated:

> *"It was found that the snack and animal food patterns were associated with a high risk of depression and anxiety, while the traditional diet pattern was associated with a low risk."*

In New Zealand, a cross-sectional population-based study[86] looked at the effect of diet on adolescent mental health from healthy eating versus unhealthy eating. Unhealthy eating behaviors included: consuming soft drinks, unhealthy snacks (for example, biscuits, potato chips and instant noodles); fried or high-fat foods (for example, french fries and pies); sweet foods (for example, chocolates and ice cream); and purchasing snacks from convenience stores. Mental health was assessed using the emotional functioning subscale of the Pediatric Quality of Life instrument. They found "significant relationships between diet quality and mental health."

---

[85] Weng, T., Hao, J., Qian, Q., Cao, H., Fu, J., Sun, Y., & ... Tao, F. (2012). Is there any relationship between dietary patterns and depression and anxiety in Chinese adolescents?. *Public Health Nutrition, 15*(4), 673-682. doi:10.1017/S1368980011003077.
[86] Kulkarni, A. A., Swinburn, B. A., & Utter, J. (2014). Associations between diet quality and mental health in socially disadvantaged New Zealand adolescents. European Journal of Clinical Nutrition Eur J Clin Nutr, 69(1), 79-83. doi:10.1038/ejcn.2014.130.

PEDIATRIC DIETARY PATTERNS AND DEPRESSION

Perhaps even more important than for adolescents, adequate nutrition for younger children is a well-known critical factor for growth and development, not only in physiological terms, but also for optimal brain and cognitive function development[87]. Inadequate nutrition has a detrimental effect on children's health and predispose to childhood obesity, dental caries, poor academic performance, emotional and behavioral difficulties.

In October 2013, results from a very large prospective cohort study of 20,000 women and their young children indicated early poor nutritional exposures in utero were related to risk for behavioral and emotional problems in their children[88]. These difficulties were more severe if the child's dietary pattern after birth was also poor.

A cross-sectional analysis of the dietary patterns of Spanish school children ages 6 – 9 was compared with the Center for Epidemiologic Studies Depression Scale for Children Questionnaire to measure depressive symptoms[89]. Their conclusion was that for children:

---

[87] Gómez-Pinilla, F. (2008). Brain foods: The effects of nutrients on brain function. Nature Reviews Neuroscience Nat Rev Neurosci, 9(7), 568-578. doi:10.1038/nrn2421.

[88] Jacka, FN, Ystrom, E, Brantsaeter, AL, Karevold, E, Roth, C, Haugen, M, Meltzer, HM, Schjolberg, S, Berk M (2013) Maternal and early postnatal nutrition and mental health of offspring by age 5 years: a prospective cohort study. Journal of the American Academy of Child & Adolescent Psychiatry 52 (9), 1038-1047.

[89] Rubio-López, N., Morales-Suárez-Varela, M., Pico, Y., Livianos-Aldana, L., & Llopis-González, A. (2016). Nutrient Intake and Depression Symptoms in Spanish Children: The ANIVA Study. International Journal of Environmental Research and Public Health IJERPH, 13(3), 352. doi:10.3390/ijerph13030352.

"Nutritional inadequacy plays an important role in mental health and poor nutrition may contribute to the pathogenesis of depression."

The mechanisms behind these effects in children and adolescents are not well described.

Beyond the obvious neurologic development in utero, we know that neurologic development continues after birth and extends throughout childhood and adolescence into young adulthood[90]. It therefore seems logical that a highly nutrient dense diet could result in an advantage in brain development with cognitive, emotional, and behavioral implications.

This could be an effect additional to the now apparent influence diet has on the mental health of adults through inflammation and the immune system, oxidative stress and neurotropic factors. Focus on psychiatric disorders in childhood and adolescence is particularly important given the fact that three quarters of lifetime psychiatric disorders will first emerge by late adolescence or early adulthood[91].

There is a multitude of reasons why judicious choice of dietary patterns is particularly important to establish early.

Therefore, in all practices of medicine, regardless of specialization, it is important to include nutritional habits in assessments of children, adolescents, and adults. Dietary advice and education enhances both physical and mental heath.

---

[90] Giedd, JN (2010) Structural MRI of pediatric brain development: what have we learned and where are we going? Neuron 67 (5), 728-34.

[91] Kessler, R. C., Berglund, P., Demler, O., Jin, R., Merikangas, K. R., & Walters, E. E. (2005). Lifetime Prevalence and Age-of-Onset Distributions of DSM-IV Disorders in the National Comorbidity Survey Replication. Archives of General Psychiatry, 62(6), 593. doi:10.1001/archpsyc.62.6.593.

FETAL

Nutritional programming during fetal development may influence the risk of chronic disease in adult life.

GERIATRIC: THE EFFECT OF DIET ON MOOD AND COGNITION

Mood disorders are a significant health care issue for the elderly and are associated with disability, decreased quality of life, functional decline, mortality from comorbid medical conditions (including suicide), demands on caregivers, and increased use of health services. An estimated 15% of all persons aged 65 and older are in need of mental health services[92].

The incidence of depression increases into our senior years[93]. A growing body of epidemiological evidence including both cross-sectional and longitudinal studies suggests a relationship between diet/nutrition and mental health at all ages but particularly so in the geriatric population. This may be a result of a number of factors but from a nutritional standpoint, older adults tend to have a decreased appetite (possibly because of decreased sensation of flavor as well as decreased activity level), poor dental status, and functional or cognitive impairments.

---

[92] US Census Bureau. Profile of General Demographic Characteristics for the United States, 2000 [table]. 2000. Available at: http://www.census.gov/pressrelease/www/2001/tables/ dp_us_2000. pdf. Accessed September 15, 2006.

[93] Williamson C (2009) Dietary factors and depression in older people. Br J Community Nurs 14, 422–426.

Strongly decreased appetite or malnutrition and depression are highly prevalent in the elderly[94] and can lead to unfavorable outcomes. In one cross-sectional study, 337 elderly subjects (193 females) were selected[95]. Depressive symptoms and nutritional status were determined by the Geriatric Depression Scale and the Mini-Nutritional Assessment questionnaires, respectively. The results revealed an association of depression with malnutrition among elderly subjects. Also, depression appeared to worsen nutritional status.

A prospective study of elderly Taiwanese utilized the Survey of Health and Living Status of the Elderly in Taiwan to measure dietary quality and the Center for Epidemiologic Studies Depression Rating Scale to measure mood states[96]. A population of over 4000 individuals was examined every 3- 4 years (1989 – 2007). Results were reported as:

> *"More frequent consumption of vegetables appears protective against depressive symptoms over time in older persons. These results have practical implications in geriatric health promotion. Older people should be encouraged to consume more vegetables since ageing is associated with a decrease in vegetable consumption."*

---

[94] Love, A. S., & Love, R. J. (2007). Depression and Diet in Elderly Community-Dwelling Mexican and European Americans. *Psychiatric Times, 24*(2), 62-63.

[95] Ahmadi, S. M., Mohammadi, M. R., Mostafavi, S., Keshavarzi, S., Kooshesh, S., Joulaei, H., & ... Lankarani, K. B. (2013). Dependence of the Geriatric Depression on Nutritional Status and Anthropometric Indices in Elderly Population. *Iranian Journal Of Psychiatry, 8*(2), 92-96.

[96] Tsai, A. C., Chang, T., & Chi, S. (2011). Frequent consumption of vegetables predicts lower risk of depression in older Taiwanese – results of a prospective population-based study. Public Health Nutr. Public Health Nutrition, 15(06), 1087-1092. doi:10.1017/s1368980011002977.

Another cross-sectional study found a high risk of malnutrition associated with depressive symptoms in older South Africans living in KwaZulu-Natal, South Africa[97].

Yet another study had the objective to examine the relationship between late-life depression and intake of fruits and vegetables[98]. The researchers hypothesized that fruit and vegetable intake would be lower in members of a depressed group compared with a non-depressed control group. All participants were over 60 years old and completed a nutrition questionnaire. This sample included patients who met *DSM-IV* diagnostic criteria for major depressive disorder as well as a comparison group without criteria for depression. Their results were:

"Intakes of fruits, vegetables, ... were found to be inversely associated with depression in this sample of elderly patients with depression."

Mild cognitive impairment is recognized now as part of a spectrum of cognitive disorders often leading to dementia. There are many factors involved in such a process (Chapters 4 – 6 will review these) – could dietary pattern be one of them?

---

[97] Naidoo, I., Charlton, K. E., Esterhuizen, T., Cassim, B., & Ester-huizen, T. M. (2015). High risk of malnutrition associated with depressive symptoms in older South Africans living in KwaZulu-Natal, South Africa: a cross-sectional survey. *Journal Of Health, Population & Nutrition*, 191-8. doi:10.1186/s41043-015-0030-0.
[98] Payne, M. E., Steck, S. E., George, R. R., & Steffens, D. C. (2012). Fruit, Vegetable, and Antioxidant Intakes Are Lower in Older Adults with Depression. *Journal Of The Academy Of Nutrition & Dietetics*, *112*(12), 2022-2027. doi:10.1016/j.jand.2012.08.026.

Adherence to a standard Mediterranean Diet and scores on the Mini-Mental State Examination, a measure of cognitive impairment, was examined for 237 elderly men and 320 women residing in Velestino, Greece (a rural Greek town[99]). The poorer the adherence to the Mediterranean Diet, the more cognitive impairment was indicated.

A cross-sectional study was performed to assess the association between unhealthy dietary habits and cognition in older adults from southern Brazil.[100] Cognition was measured by the Mini-Mental State Examination. Unhealthy dietary patterns were grouped by low intake of fruits and vegetables (four servings/day); fish (< 1 serving/week); and habitual fatty meat intake (yes/no). Adjustments were made for age, education level, income, smoking status, alcohol intake, leisure-time physical activity, depression symptoms, chronic diseases, and body mass index. Their conclusion:

"Regular intake of fruits, vegetables, and fish in exchange of fatty meats may be a viable public policy strategy to preserve cognition in aging."

The Mediterranean Diet was explored as a means to slow cognitive decline and decrease the risk of dementia in a review of ten prospective cohort studies and one cross-sectional study[101]. Results were:

---

[99] Katsiardanis, K., Diamantaras, A., Dessypris, N., Michelakos, T., Anastasiou, A., Katsiardani, K., & ... Petridou, E. T. (2013). Cognitive Impairment and Dietary Habits Among Elders: The Velestino Study. *Journal Of Medicinal Food*, *16*(4), 343-350. doi:10.1089/jmf.2012.0225.

[100] França, V. F., Barbosa, A. R., & D'Orsi, E. (2016). Cognition and Indicators of Dietary Habits in Older Adults from Southern Brazil. *Plos ONE*, *11*(2), 1-12. doi:10.1371/journal.pone.0147820.

[101] Opie, R. S., Ralston, R. A., & Walker, K. Z. (2013). Adherence to a Mediterranean-style diet can slow the rate of cognitive decline and de-

"There is strong evidence for the protective role of a Mediterranean-style diet against cognitive decline and development of Alzheimer's disease."

In the next chapter we shall delve deeper into the neuropsychiatric explanation for these epidemiologic findings.

> ***The prevalence of mental disorders is high and associated with dietary patterns. Fruit and vegetables appear to be protective, while processed foods and animal products increase the risk for mood disorders.***

crease the risk of dementia: a systematic review. *Nutrition & Dietetics*, *70*(3), 206-217. doi:10.1111/1747-0080.12016.

CHAPTER 4

Cerebrovascular Disease

"Whatever is good for the goose is good for the gander[102]."

When thinking of vascular disease, cardiovascular disease usually comes immediately to mind. After all, it is the number one cause of death in the United States and many other Western civilizations[103]. Miraculously, and unappreciated, there are a number of excellent research studies[104] [105] [106] that

---

[102] From earlier "what's sauce for the goose is sauce for the gander" (1670s). Other early forms include "as deep drinketh the goose as the gander" (1562); John Heywood, The Proverbs, Epigrams, and Miscellanies of John Heywood, 1562, p. 82.

[103] Xu J, Murphy SL, Kochanek KD, et al: Deaths: Final Data for 2013. Natl Vital Stat Rep 2016;64:1-119.

[104] Ornish, D., Brown, S., Billings, J., Scherwitz, L., Armstrong, W., Ports, T., . . . Brand, R. (1990). Can lifestyle changes reverse coronary heart disease? The Lancet,336(8708), 129-133. doi:10.1016/0140-6736(90)91656-u.

indicate heart disease is not only quite preventable but *reversible* through a diet rich in plants and lower in processed foods and animal products.

But the arteries that become damaged in the heart are quite similar to the arteries that serve all our organs, including that most delicate and sensitive of all - the brain, resulting in cerebrovascular disease, the second leading cause of death worldwide[107]. Given the similarity of cardiovascular and cerebrovascular disease mechanisms, it is not surprising that there is a close association between depression and cardiovascular disease[108].

Well before cerebrovascular disease results in death, there is often a gradual deterioration in the tissue served by the very high degree of vascularization in the brain, neurons being much more sensitive to oxygen deprivation than other types of cells. Even small otherwise unnoticeable damage to the brain can have life changing effects on our cognition, emotions, and behavior.

---

[105] Ornish, D. (1998). Intensive Lifestyle Changes for Reversal of Coronary Heart Disease. *Jama, 280*(23), 2001. doi:10.1001/ jama.280.23.2001.

[106] Esselstyn, C. B. (1999). Updating a 12-year experience with arrest and reversal therapy for coronary heart disease (an overdue requiem for palliative cardiology). *The American Journal of Cardiology, 84*(3), 339-341. doi:10.1016/s0002-9149(99)00290-8.

[107] Ward, Helen; Toledano, Mireille B.; Shaddick, Gavin; Davies, Bethan; Elliott, Paul (2012-05-24). *Oxford Handbook of Epidemiology for Clinicians*. OUP Oxford. p. 310.

[108] Nemeroff, C. B., & Goldschmidt-Clermont, P. J. (2012). Heartache and heartbreak—the link between depression and cardiovascular disease. *Nat Rev Cardiol Nature Reviews Cardiology, 9*(9), 526-539. doi:10.1038/nrcardio.2012.91.

So is it likely that cerebrovascular disease, like cardiovascular disease, is preventable and in some regard possibly even reversible, too?

In this chapter, we will explain the cause and effect of cerebrovascular disease, its similarities and differences from cardiovascular disease and how it affects mental wellness. Finally, we shall describe how to make life style changes to avoid and possibly reverse the effects of cerebrovascular illness.

NUTRIENT DELIVERY – THE CIRCULATORY SYSTEM

One of the simplest – and most vital – processes of the body is the delivery of nutrients, including oxygen and water, to each cell in the body. Interruption of this delivery process for more than a few minutes can lead to cell death. We say simplest because, after all, the circulatory system consists of basically a pump (the heart) and a bunch of pipes (the blood vessels). From a mechanical standpoint, the pump should not stop and the pipes should not get clogged.

If the heart pump stops altogether, there is system shutdown known as "clinical death[109]" that typically leads to "legal death" without heroic measures being taken. However, if a single blood vessel gets partially or completely clogged, there may only be a penalty, infarction and cell death, in the area served by those vessels. If that penalized area happens to be part of the heart itself and a significant volume or location of the heart,

---

[109] "Clinical death" is the medical term for cessation of blood flow and occurs when the heart stops beating, a condition called cardiac arrest. Halting of blood circulation had been historically irreversible and the definition of "death" but with the invention of cardiopulmonary resuscitation, defibrillation, epinephrine injection, and other treatments, the absence of blood circulation has come to be called clinical death to reflect the possibility of post-arrest resuscitation.

however, this could be particularly problematic because the heart is a critical element in the circulation. This is why there is so much attention to even partial narrowing of the cross-sectional area available for blood flow in the coronary arteries serving the heart.

In the case of the development of partial narrowing of areas of the heart resulting in reduced flow of oxygen and nutrients, there may be temporary chest pain, or "stable" angina, associated with physical exertion. This can serve as a warning signal to reduce the level of exertion so that more serious irreversible damage does not occur. Some other areas of the body experience the effects of intermittent nutrient demand beyond the capability of the delivery supply due to blockages of the vessel conduit – for example "claudication" in the extremities that similarly reflect this situation with notification through pain. However, most organs do not have this warning system.

This is unfortunate because one of those other organs is more sensitive to stoppage of the flow of nutrients than all others: the brain. In fact, when "clinical death" occurs, the heart has stopped but no organs are actually "dead"; consciousness ceases in about 15 seconds due to lack of blood perfusion and brain injury begins within about three minutes. Actual "brain death" – usually the determining factor in "legal death" happens somewhat more gradually, but certainly catastrophic injury or brain death can take place in about ten minutes without blood circulation in the brain.

Most tissues and organs of the body can survive clinical death for considerable periods. The heart itself could survive up to 20 – 30 minutes[110]. Blood circulation can be stopped in the entire body below the heart for at least 30 minutes. Severed limbs

---

110 http://heartfoundation2009.com/miocardial-infarction.

may be successfully reattached after six hours of no blood circulation, and bone, tendon, and skin can survive as long as 8 to 12 hours[111].

So the most sensitive organ to oxygen deprivation and other nutrient transfer is not the heart- it is the brain, and it does not give us warning signs when it is in the process of developing serious blockages in blood circulation, having no pain receptors. With 100,000 miles of circulatory vessels in the brain, there are lots of opportunities for localized "traffic jams" of blood flow.

Although the potential problem of narrowing and closure of circulatory conduits extends to all areas of the body, we shall focus on the brain.

THE "SACRED DISEASE"

> *"I am about to discuss the disease called "sacred'. It is not, in my opinion, any more divine or more sacred than other diseases, but has a natural cause. The fact is that the cause of this affliction is the brain. These things we suffer all come from the brain, when it is not healthy."*
> *~Hippocrates, circa 400 BCE*

Perhaps the most impressive accomplishment of the Hippocratic epoch was to attempt to rationally explain individual diseases without recourse to magical or religious interpretations. The "sacred disease" was so named prior to Hippocrates because of the profound presentation: individuals were suddenly "struck" down dead as if from lightning, but

---

111 Replantation , Author: Mark I Langdorf, MD, MHPE, FAAEM, FACEP, RDMS; Chief Editor: Rick Kulkarni, MD; http://emedicine. medscape.com/ article/827648-overview.

there being no lightning present, this had been interpreted as accomplished by the hand of God. As Cooke wrote in 1820[112]:

"A disease in which the patient falls to the ground, often suddenly, and lies without sense or voluntary motion. Persons, instantaneously thus affected, as if struck by lightning; were, by the ancients, denominated, attoniti aut, syderati (struck by lightning; tempest)."

We still refer to this phenomenon as a "stroke" as if the victim was struck down by some unknown force. But now we know the source can be a number of causes, including vessel occlusion as indicated above or by a hemorrhagic cerebrovascular accident in which vessels in the brain burst, typically from high blood pressure and a weakened vessel wall. Purists would substitute "disease" (or "event") for "accident," presumably removing an assumption of causality; an "accident" being reserved for an incident that happens unintentionally to us, for example from a crushing blow to the head caused by someone else. As we shall see, most of these stroke events indeed occur not by accident but can be avoided by proper lifestyle choices.

We shall use "stroke" interchangeably with cerebrovascular event to refer to brain injury caused by any disruption of blood supply to the brain, whether it be from vessel hemorrhage (hemorrhagic stroke) or from vessel occlusion (ischemic stroke).

Shockingly, strokes are the leading cause of adult disability in the United States and Europe, and together with associated dementia, are the leading cause of death worldwide[113].

---

[112] Cooke J (1820) A treatise on nervous diseases, p 157. Longman, Hurst, Rees, Orme and Brown. London.

It is perhaps motivating to learn of these disease processes as they were discovered historically. Credit for having been the first to propose that occlusion of a vessel might result in a stroke is generally assigned to Gregor Nymann (1594-1638) of Wittenberg, Germany[114]. However, the occlusion was thought to be of "humoral flow" rather than that of blood circulation and "bloodletting" was still a treatment of choice.

The English pathologist Matthew Baillie, in 1793, had specifically referred to diseased arteries of the elderly brain in the final chapter of his Morbid Anatomy on "Diseased appearances of the brain and its mechanisms[115]". The diseased arteries he had conclusively related to the occurrence of intracerebral hemorrhage. He also described:

> *"bony or earthy matter being deposited in the coats of the arteries, by which they lose a part of their contractile and distensible powers, as well as of their tenacity,"*

and went on to reason[116]:

> *"The vessels of the brain under such circumstances of disease are much more liable to be ruptured than in a healthy state. Whenever blood is accumulated in unusual*

---

[113] Feigin VL (2005). "Stroke epidemiology in the developing world". Lancet 365 (9478): 2160–1.

[114] McHenry LC, Jr. (1969). Garrison's History of Neurology, Charles C. Thomas. Springfield, Il.

[115] Baillie M (1793). The Morbid Anatomy of Some of the Most Important Parts of the Human Body., J. Johnson and
   G. Nicol, London.

[116] McHenry LC, Jr. (1969). Garrison's History of Neurology., Charles C. Thomas. Springfield, IL, p 130.

> *quantity, or the circulation is going on in them
> with unusual vigor, they are liable to this
> accident, and accordingly in either of these
> states ruptures frequently happen."*

Of course the etiology of these phenomena was completely unknown. It was Rudolf Virchow (1821- 1902), a mid-19th century German pathologist, who would advance the vascular theories of occlusive stroke with the introduction of the terms "thrombosis" and "embolus" into the medical literature[117]. Virchow noted that thrombosis (a clot) could occur, not as the result of an inflammatory process, as was generally thought at this time, but rather because of some pathologic process in the artery or arteriole. An inflammatory response followed and therefore was a secondary event. Virchow in 1847[118] also proposed an alternate means of vessel occlusion, a process he called "embolism":

> *"Here there is either no essential change in the
> vessel wall and its surroundings, or this is
> ostensibly secondary. I feel perfectly justified in
> claiming that these clots never originated in the
> local circulation but that they are tom off at a
> distance and carried along in the blood stream
> as far as they can go."*

So the vascular origins of stroke were mechanistically described by mid-19th century, but the phrase cerebrovascular disease and an understanding of its true nature as a vascular disease entity is relatively new. It was first listed in the 8th edition of the International Classification of Disease (ICD-8) in 1965,

---

[117] Schiller I' (1970). Concepts of stroke before and after Virchow. Med Hist 14: 115-131.

[118] Ibid, p 127.

where it was included under "diseases of the circulation," distinct from diseases of the nervous system.

To summarize, there are two main types of cerebrovascular diseases: ischemic disorders and hemorrhagic disorders. The former class of ischemic disorder in which blood flow to areas of the brain is blocked accounts for about 80 - 85% of patients with symptomatic cerebrovascular disease and hemorrhagic stroke in which blood flows outside of the brain vessels into surrounding tissue accounts for the other 15 to 20% of symptomatic disease[119]. Both types of diseases can lead to physical, behavioral, emotional, and cognitive changes and both types of diseases are largely preventable by proper lifestyle choices.

The ischemic disorders all start with the atherosclerotic process, and that process begins with excessive blood cholesterol.

ATHEROSCLEROSIS[120]

The process of artery clogging or "hardening" is known as atherosclerosis[121], from the Greek *arteria* meaning artery and *sclerosis*, meaning hardness. By the way, the other half of the

---

[119] Robinson, R. G. (1998). *The clinical neuropsychiatry of stroke: cognitive, behavioral and emotional disorders following vascular brain injury* p. 36. Cambridge University Press.

[120] The following terms are similar, yet distinct, in both spelling and meaning, and can be easily confused: arteriosclerosis, arteriolosclerosis, and atherosclerosis. Arteriosclerosis is a general term describing any hardening (and loss of elasticity) of medium or large arteries (arteriolosclerosis is any hardening (and loss of elasticity) of arterioles (small arteries); atherosclerosis is a hardening of an artery specifically due to an atheromatous plaque. The term atherogenic is used for substances or processes that cause atherosclerosis.

[121] Aldons J. Lusis (14 September 2000). "Atherosclerosis". Nature 407 (6801): 233–241.

circulatory system consisting of veins does not become clogged by the process described here because of the lower pressure in the venous blood returning to the heart and therefore smaller shear stresses, the different composition of the vein wall, and the different nutrient content, primarily oxygen level[122]. Again, just for emphasis, these arterial vessels occur throughout the body – such as the head and brain that are of particular interest here – not just the heart.

The human brain uses 20% of the body's energy but is only 2% of the body's weight.

Our understanding of atherosclerosis has increased dramatically rather recently as a result of new research techniques such as using ultrasound within individual arteries so we can "look through" the walls of these vessels. It turns out that this disease process begins a lot earlier in life than we thought; studies have shown that nearly all children in the United States have at least the precursor of atherosclerosis by age ten[123].

ANATOMY OF CEREBROVASCULAR DISEASE

An artery cross section consists of three parts: the innermost layer is called the epithelium and is only one single cell thick; the middle layer is composed primarily of muscle fibers that allow the artery to dilate or constrict; the outermost layer is connective tissue.

The building blocks for the atherosclerotic process are LDL (low-density lipoprotein) and cholesterol. The LDL is essentially a

---

[122] The exceptions are the four pulmonary veins in which oxygenated blood returns to the heart via the left atrium.

[123] Voller, R. D., & Strong, W. B. (1981). Pediatric aspects of athero-sclerosis. *American Heart Journal, 101*(6), 815-836. doi:10.1016/0002-8703(81)90621-9.

transport vehicle for cholesterol, a steroid necessary for cell membranes and certain hormone production, so the entire atherosclerotic process is dependent on *excessive cholesterol*. The problem begins when certain small LDL particles (so called Pattern B[124]) find their way between the epithelial cells into the middle layer of the cell wall. Once in this middle layer, the cholesterol-laden LDL can become oxidized by free radicals resulting in a toxic product. This toxin triggers an inflammatory process in which white blood cells also pass through the endothelium into the middle cell layer.

As the white blood cells undergo some changes (and a new name: macrophages), they engulf the cholesterol-rich oxidized LDL and change form and name once again, becoming foam cells. These foam cells are rather short lived as well, dying and releasing their lipid content, creating what is called a lipid core. A fibrous cap consisting of collagen and elastin forms over the lipid core in an attempt by the body to heal itself. This fat-pus gruel is called an atheroma (from the Greek ἀθήρωμα "lump of gruel") or atherosclerotic plaque.

We now know that atherosclerotic plaques develop and progress in the artery wall long before they begin the encroachment on the interior diameter, or lumen, of the artery. This is because of a compensatory external diameter enlargement by the arterial wall. This is important to note for two reasons: first, typical testing such as stress tests and angiography do not detect these plaques and, second, these early plaques are more apt to rupture than those that protrude into the lumen. It is the rupturing that causes heart attacks and strokes.

---

[124] Superko HR, Nejedly M, Garrett B (2002). "Small LDL and its clinical importance as a new CAD risk factor: a female case study". Progress in Cardiovascular Nursing 17 (4): 167–73.

Plaques prone to rupture include those of a large lipid core covered by a thin fibrous cap. When the plaque ruptures through the endothelial wall into the lumen of the artery, the lipid core comes into direct contact with the blood. This sets the stage for the formation of a clot or thrombus. The thrombus may partially or totally block an artery, causing a gradual or sudden reduction in blood flow. Partial blockage of coronary arteries may present with the symptoms of angina pain in the heart or transient ischemic attacks (TIAs) in the brain. Gripping heart pain is obvious; TIAs may be symptomatic or completely unnoticed. Complete blockage of the lumen over a long enough time interval will result in cell death downstream of the blocked blood flow; in the case of the coronary artery this is termed a myocardial infarction or commonly as a "heart attack". In the brain, there is cerebral infarction or a "stroke".

In stable angina, the developing atheroma is protected with a fibrous cap. This cap (atherosclerotic plaque) may rupture in unstable angina, allowing blood clots to precipitate and further decrease the lumen of the coronary vessel.

As the burden of plaque build-up continues, the artery can no longer compensate sufficiently and the plaque begins to protrude into the lumen. This generally happens when the plaque reaches 40% of the vessel circumference. Naturally, a combination of these protrusions and newly forming thrombi are particularly dangerous.

More often than not, the newly formed thrombi detach, moving into the circulation and eventually occlude smaller downstream arterial branches, a so-called thromboembolism. When this happens in the brain, it is called a cerebral embolism type of ischemic infarction or stroke.

IT'S THE CHOLESTEROL

In a 2010 editorial in the American Journal of Cardiology titled "It's the Cholesterol Stupid," the editor of that journal for the previous thirty years and the executive director of the Baylor Heart and Vascular Institute William Roberts, MD, stated that elevated cholesterol is the cause of atherosclerosis and offered these facts:

> *"Atherosclerotic plaques are easily produced experimentally in herbivores simply by feeding these animals cholesterol (e.g., egg yolks) or saturated fats. Indeed, atherosclerosis is probably the second easiest disease to produce experimentally.*
>
> o *Cholesterol is present in atherosclerotic plaques in experimentally produced atherosclerosis and in plaques in human beings.*
>
> o *Societies and subjects with high serum cholesterol levels (total and low-density lipoprotein [LDL] cholesterol) compared to populations and subjects with low levels have a high frequency of atherosclerotic events, a high frequency of dying from these events, and a large quantity (burden) of plaque in their arteries*[125].

---

[125] Kromhout, D., Menotti, A., Bloemberg, B., Aravanis, C., Blackburn, H., Buzina, R., . . . Toshima, H. (1995). Dietary Saturated and transFatty Acids and Cholesterol and 25-Year Mortality from Coronary Heart Disease: The Seven Countries Study. *Preventive Medicine, 24*(3), 308-315. doi:10.1006/pmed.1995.1049.

○ ***Lowering total and LDL cholesterol levels decrease the frequency of atherosclerotic events, the chances of dying from these events, and the quantity of plaques in the arteries. "***

It deserves restating that the *only* way to produce atherosclerotic plaques is to give animal products to a herbivore, such as a human (we have evolved to accept a variety of foodstuffs to survive but as primates we have been herbivores for 85 million years – refer to our book *The New Ancestral Diet*[126]). One cannot produce these plaques in a carnivore.

Atherosclerotic disease is caused by excess cholesterol in the diet, as occurs from a diet of animals and animal products.

Dr. Roberts goes on to say that although there are risk factors for introduction and propagation of plaques such as increased blood pressure, diabetes or obesity, inactivity, and cigarette smoking, it is *necessary* to have an elevated LDL cholesterol (greater than 60 mg/ dl or serum total cholesterol greater than 150 mg/dl) or there will be no atherosclerotic plaques.

Because there is no cholesterol in plants, only animals chemically manufacture it, the way to lower your cholesterol is to eat only plants, no animal products.

---

[126] Aiken, R.C., and Aiken, D.C. (2015) *The new ancestral diet*. Go Ahead Publishing, Los Angeles, California.

CEREBROVASCULAR DISEASE AND DEPRESSION

For more than 100 years, clinicians have recognized that emotional disorders accompany stroke[127]. While it is still generally unknown why this is true, there are at least three lines of reasoning. The first is simply that an emotional disorder is an understandable psychological response to stress that results from other physical manifestations post stroke; another is that there is some pathophysiological process that the brain goes through after injury that somehow leads to clinical depression. The third is a result of the low level chronic inflammation following macro, mini, or even micro-strokes; more on that in the next chapter.

The brain is more sensitive to vascular disease than the heart.

As noted previously, strokes had been considered a medical condition to be diagnosed and treated primarily by the neurologist until about 1965, with ICD-8 and the recognition of the origin to be vascular and therefore a condition to be shared with other medical specialties such as internal medicine and vascular surgery.

Nevertheless, the most controversial areas of research in post stroke mood disorders have to do with "lesion location"[128], the neurological approach.

A simple but classic example of how a neurologist goes about "finding the lesion", or the source of a problem, was the presentation in 1861 of Monsieur Leborgne's loss of speech but

---

[127] Robinson, R. G. (1998). *The clinical neuropsychiatry of stroke: cognitive, behavioral and emotional disorders following vascular brain injury* p. 15. Cambridge University Press.

[128] Ibid, p. 94.

not loss of comprehension or mental function. He was nicknamed "Tan" due to his inability to clearly speak any words other than "tan". When French physician, surgeon, and anatomist Pierre Paul Broca learned of this patient, he traveled to see him but as fortune would have it, M. Leborgne had just passed. Dr. Broca proceeded with an autopsy and found that "the lesion" was "within the third convolution of the left frontal lobe", an area of the brain now called "Broca's Area"[129] and the condition termed "aphasia" (the brains of many of Broca's aphasic patients are still preserved in the Musée Dupuytren in Paris).

Early attempts at lesion location for the "neurotic or distracted" patient yielded a few interesting, if uncommon and odd, case descriptions. The famous neurologist Joseph Babinski in 1914 described stroke patients with a right hemispheric lesion who were indifferent to their impairments and in fact inappropriately cheerful about them[130]. Another example of lesion-specific emotional behavior is that of pathologic laughter or crying without apparent triggers; Ironside in 1956 associated this unusual condition with strokes of an area of the brainstem called the pons (producing "pseudobulbar palsy[131]").

SHOW ME THE LESION

As previously mentioned, the first purveyors of medicine could be thought of as "psychiatrists" in that it began "when one man attempted to relieve another man's suffering by influencing

---

[129] Broca, Paul. "Remarks on the Seat of the Faculty of Articulated Language, Following an Observation of Aphemia (Loss of Speech)". Bulletin de la Société Anatomique, Vol. 6, (1861), 330–357.

[130] This condition is called "anosognosia" after Babinski, J., "Contribution a l'etude des trobles mentaux dans l'hemiplegie organique cerbrale (anosognosie). Rev Neurol (Paris) 27:845-8, 1914.

[131] Ironside, R., Disorders of laughter due to brain leisons. Brain 75:589-609, 1956.

him"[132]. These "influences" have primarily been psychological until well into the twentieth century. Once identifiable physiologic etiologies began to emerge for many pathologic conditions, this provided a dilemma for the emerging field of psychiatry as there were no identifiable "lesions"or otherwise clear causative factors.

Enter Sigismund Schlomo Freud, an Austrian neurologist, born in 1856. The inability to locate an anatomical basis for emotion perhaps influenced Freud to propose abstract theories of "the mind" as opposed to "the body". Thus psychoanalytic theory and "talk therapy" was born. Freud further abstracted the mind into the conscious and unconscious, neither with direct biological correlates, which eventually fell into disrepute among most contemporary psychiatrists.

So note that the ancient healers merged mind-body-spirit into basically one entity with emphasis on the spirit; the Greek physicians separated out the spirit part; with emerging technology of the nineteenth century the body was emphasized apart from the problematic complexities of "the mind". Thus the mind-body-spirit triad was dissected.

Psychiatry is one of the five basic areas of medicine taught in all medical schools (the other four being internal medicine, surgery, pediatrics, and obstetrics/ gynecology – note neurology is not amongst these). This is becasue the emotionally/ behaviorally disordered patient group is large and problematic. A portion of this group over the past hundred years or so have in fact been found to have identifiable "lesions" or organic causes of their psychiatric presentation leaving the remainder for the subjective art of classification merely based on emotional and behavioral symptoms but

---

[132] Papowitz, E. B. (1973). Discussion. The American Journal of Psychoanalysis, 33(2), 163-166. doi:10.1007/bf01872572.

without a clear etiology. In fact, once there is a clear biological explanation for the presentation of the disorder, it is then referred to one of the other specialties or subspecialties of medicine.

DIFFERENT STROKES FOR DIFFERENT FOLKS

This rather confusing specialty ownership of disorders that involve physiological changes yet have emotional, behavioral and cognitive effects is illustrated nicely by strokes. The approach of the psychiatrist frequently is to treat psychiatric symptoms with the same psychotropic medications and psychotherapy regardless of the etiology because in the vast majority of cases there is no known etiology.

Academic or not, there has been a known association of strokes and mental disorder since at least the time of a founder of "modern psychiatry", Emil Kraepelin[133], who wrote in 1921:

> *"The diagnosis of states of depression may, apart from the distinctions discussed, offer difficulties especially when the possibility of atherosclerosis has to be taken into consideration. It may, at a time, be an accompanying phenomenon of manic depression insanity but at another time may itself engender states of depression."*

Ulman and Greun as early as 1960[134]noted that not only are post-stroke physical and cognitive limitations stressful, also the

[133] Kraepelin, E., (1921). *Manic depressive insanity and paranoia*, Edinburgh: E & S Livingston.
[134] Ullman, M., & Gruen, A. (1961). Behavioral Changes In Patients With Strokes. American Journal of Psychiatry, 117(11), 1004-1009. doi:10.1176/ajp.117.11.1004.

various coping mechanisms one might possess are potentially injury-compromised, rendering emotional recovery more challenging, this devoid of any other and additional neurophysiologic mechanisms leading to mood disorder.

While there may be a direct effect from the removal of discrete areas of the brain injured by stroke, it appears emotional, behavioral, and cognitive decline post injury is much more complex than associated localized injury but instead affected by areas of the brain that are not directly injured but influenced by lack of "activation" or "inhibition" signals from the diseased regions.

We know that strokes can cause a range of emotional and personality changes in a person through death of sections of the brain, that is apart from the stressful effects of having suffered a stroke and the potential physical disabilities that might result.[135] Some of these changes can appear as clinical depression. Overall prevalence rates of depression in clinical stroke victims has been estimated to be about 20%.[136] We know that depression from strokes involving the left side of the brain is particularly severe and this severity increases with frontal lobe involvement.[137] This makes sense from our

---

[135] This was first described in 1977 in an interesting study of disability matched stroke and orthopedic control groups, reducing the environmental factor of disability from the statistics; Folstein MF, Maiberger R, McHugh PR: Mood disorder as a specific complication of stroke. J Neurol Neurosurg Psychiatry 1977; 40:1018–1020.

[136] Robinson, R. G. (2003). Poststroke depression: Prevalence, diagnosis, treatment, and disease progression. Biological Psychiatry, 54(3), 376-387. doi:10.1016/s0006-3223(03)00423-2.

[137] And of the frontal lobe, part of the prefrontal cortex called the ventromedial cortex is particularly involved and has dense connections to the emotional circuit of the brain called the limbic system. Narushima, K., Kosier, J. T., & Robinson, R. G. (2003). A Reappraisal of Poststroke Depression, Intra- and Inter-Hemispheric Lesion Location Using Meta-

understanding of the association of the left front area of the brain with positive emotions and motivation, so an injury to that area can be thought to simply compromise its function.

"SILENT" CEREBRAL INFARCTION AND MOOD

Thus far we have been discussing cerebrovascular diseases that are symptomatic. However, most disease processes are either asymptomatic or subtle and gradual in their effect on emotion, behavior and cognition, the higher integrative aspects of brain function.

Usually when one thinks of strokes one thinks of physical limitations, that is of difficulties such as with speech and movement but that is just the tip of the iceberg or just the lateral outer surface of the motor cortex.

A study in 1998 estimated that more than 11 million people experienced silent strokes in the United States[138]. A "silent" stroke is simply one for which you are unaware. Usually you are unaware because either it involved a small area of the brain or it involved an area of the brain that had no discernable effect on your senses or observable behavior.

The brain executes its various functions as an integrated entity through connective pathways of various brain regions. The complex function of emotion or specifically mood involves many brain regions connected by what often is termed the "serotonin pathway" because the neurotransmitter serotonin is quite active in this messaging.

Analysis. The Journal of Neuropsychiatry and Clinical Neurosciences, 15(4), 422-430. doi:10.1176/jnp.15.4.422.

[138] Leary, M. C., & Saver, J. L. (2003). Annual Incidence of First Silent Stroke in the United States: A Preliminary Estimate. Cerebrovascular Diseases, 16(3), 280-285. doi:10.1159/000071128.

A silent stroke can erode a little part of that mood pathway. After a number of silent strokes, there can be a cumulative disruptive effect that becomes clinically evident with obvious changes in mood, behavior, memory and cognition. This noticeable cumulative effect often takes some years.

In one remarkable study of elderly patients diagnosed with major depression, silent cerebral infarction was observed in 66% of those with depression onset before the age of 65 and in 94% of those with onset of depression after age 65.[139] A characteristic cognitive pattern with prominent memory deficits sometimes so severe as to suggest a "pseudo dementia" in depressed patients with vascular disease, a so called "vascular depression", has been described but this has been challenged[140].

If these silent strokes have been extensive, we generally recognize this state as "vascular dementia" with all the extreme moods, behaviors, memory and cognitive compromise associated with it. Unfortunately, this state of being is quite common; in fact, the second most common cause of dementia in the United States next to Alzheimer's disease.

---

[139] Fujikawa, T., Yamawaki, S., & Touhouda, Y. (1993). Incidence of silent cerebral infarction in patients with major depression. Stroke, 24(11), 1631-1634. doi:10.1161/01.str.24.11.1631.

[140] Vascular depressedion was first described by Alexopoulos GS, Meyers BS, Young RC, Kakuma T, Silbersweig D, Charlson M: Clinically defined vascular depression. Am J Psychiatry 1997; 154:562–565; it has been challenged by a number of more recent studies including Aben I, Lodder J, Honig A, Lousberg R, Boreas A, Verhey F: Focal or generalized vascular brain damage and vulnerability to depression after stroke: a 1-year prospective follow-up study. Int Psychogeriatr 2006; 18:19–35 and Rainer MK, Mucke HA, Zehetmayer S, Krampla W, Kuselbauer T, Weissgram S, Jungwirth S, Tragl KH, Fischer P: Data from the VITA Study do not support the concept of vascular depression. Am J Geriatr Psychiatry 2006; 14:531–537.

So there is a spectrum of presentations of this phenomenon ranging from "silent", without apparent effect at all, to complete incapacitating dementia and accompanying psychiatric disorders including depression, even psychotic states. As there is actual brain damage involved, one can understand why it is very difficult, if not impossible, to treat, for example with anti-depressants or anti-psychotic medications. Recall that the causative factor here is typically the creation and disruption of atherosclerotic plaques from excessive cholesterol in the diet.

To summarize this section on strokes, those either acutely obvious or insidious and accumulative, there is a clear mechanistic casual explanation between cerebrovascular disease and depression. But there is a lot more to the story.

BLOOD PRESSURE

The highest risk factor for death *in the world* is high blood pressure[141], contributing to nine million deaths world-wide every year[142]. This higher than expected magnitude of risk is not only a result of hemorrhagic stroke but also aneurysms, heart attacks, heart failure, and kidney failure.

---

[141] Bromfield, S., & Muntner, P. (2013). High Blood Pressure: The Leading Global Burden of Disease Risk Factor and the Need for World-wide Prevention Programs. *Current Hypertension Reports, 15*(3), 134-136. doi:10.1007/s11906-013-0340-9.

[142] S. Lim S, Vos T, Blyth F, et al. A comparative risk assessment of burden of disease and injury attributable to 67 risk factors and risk factor clusters in 21 regions, 1990-2010: a systematic analysis for the Global Burden of Disease Study 2010. *Lancet* [serial online]. December 15, 2012;380(9859):2224-2260. Available from: Academic Search Complete, Ipswich, MA. Accessed October 2, 2016.

NOT WORTH OUR SALT

Excessive sodium intake appears to be the largest contributor to high blood pressure. The mechanism is osmosis, the tendency of solutes such as sodium in the blood when in higher concentrations relative to cellular sodium to draw water into the interior of the artery. This produces a strain on the artery

> *High blood pressure, the highest risk factor for death in the world, can occur from salt in diet.*

walls; with time they become stronger and thicker, reducing their ability to expand. This translates to higher blood pressure. Unfortunately, this is a cumulative effect that worsens with age.

NON-INFARCTION CEREBROVASCULAR DISEASE AND DEPRESSION

Certain types of magnetic resonance imaging of the brain show scan hyperintensities in the white or gray matter. They are associated with affective disorders such as depression and bipolar disorder[143]. While there appears to be a clear association with cerebrovascular disease, the relation does not

> *Cerebrovascular disease is insidious and results in gradual or abrupt cognitive and emotional changes.*

appear in all cases to be simple infarction but also other etiologies such as demyelination caused by reduced local blood flow.

---

[143] Kempton, M.J., Geddes, J.R, Ettinger, U. et al. (2008). "Meta-analysis, Database, and Meta-regression of 98 Structural Imaging Studies in Bipolar Disorder," Archives of General Psychiatry, 65:1017–1032.

Another link between cerebrovascular disease and depression is suggested by the "homocysteine hypothesis"[144]. Homocysteine is an amino acid not directly obtained from your diet but manufactured by ingested methionine found in meat, eggs, cheese, and poultry and is toxic to neurons and blood vessels. It's generally recognized as a vascular risk factor along with high cholesterol, high triglycerides, diabetes, hypertension, and tobacco use[145], but underappreciated for its neurotoxicity and association with depression[146]. Deficiencies of the vitamins folic acid (B9), pyridoxine (B6), or B12 (cobalamin) can lead to high homocysteine levels.[147] Elevations of homocysteine also occur from a rather common genetic trait.[148]

Methionine, found in dietary meat products, is used in the manufacture of homocysteine in our bodies, toxic to neurons and blood vessels.

---

[144] Marshal Folstein, Timothy Liu, Inga Peter, Jennifer Buel, Lisa Arsenault, Tammy Scott, and Wendy W. Qiu, The Homocysteine Hypothesis of Depression, Am J Psychiatry, Jun 2007; 164: 861 - 867.

[145] Selhub, J. (1999). "Homocysteine metabolism.". Annual Review of Nutrition 19: 217–246.

[146] Homocysteine is toxic to neurons and blood vessels and can casue DNA breakage and oxidative stress. Mattson MP, Shea TB: Folate and homocysteine metabolism in neural plasticity and neurodegenerative disorders. Trends Neurosci 2003; 26:137–146.

[147] Miller JW, Nadeau MR, Smith D and Selhub J (1994). "Vitamin B-6 deficiency vs folate deficiency: comparison of responses to methionine loading in rats". American Journal of Clinical Nutrition 59 (5): 1033–1039.

[148] Elevations are caused by the methylene-tetrahydrofolate-reductase polymorphism genetic traits in about 10% of the world population and linked to an increased incidence of thrombosis and cardiovascular disease; Schneider JA, Rees DC, Liu YT, Clegg JB (May 1998). "Worldwide distribution of a common methylenetetrahydrofolate reductase mutation". Am. J. Hum. Genet. 62 (5): 1258–60.

The idea behind the homocysteine hypothesis is that homocysteine might cause a type of clinical depression through chemical pathways that reduce the concentrations of neurotransmitters involved with mood[149], but these studies are rather indirect, speculative, and correlative.

ALZHEIMER'S DISEASE

Alzheimer's disease is an insidious illness that begins well before any clinically evident indications. It is a neurodegenerative disorder that is not localized in the brain, like a stroke, but can affect the entire brain. Like stroke, those neurons that die as a result of the illness cannot be regenerated so the damage is irreversible. However, the disease *process* can be slowed, possibly radically.

Besides memory loss, Alzheimer's patients show dramatic personality changes, emotional and behavioral changes, disorientation, declining physical coordination, and an inability to care for themselves. Practically any psychiatric condition can be included in the presentation of the Alzheimer's patient, from depression to psychosis. Common reasons for admission to psychiatric hospitals include delusions and hallucinations accompanying assaultive behavior. In the final stages, victims are bedridden and ultimately die from infections such as pneumonia, bedsores or urinary tract infections.

---

[149] Tang HZ: [The changes of monoamine metabolites in CSF of patients with cerebral stroke]. Zhonghua Shen Jing Jing Shen Ke Za Zhi 1991; 24:130–132, 186; see also Bryer JB, Starkstein SE, Votypka V, Parikh RM, Price TR, Robinson RG: Reduction of CSF monoamine metabolites in poststroke depression: a preliminary report. J Neuropsychiatry Clin Neurosci 1992; 4:440–442 and Bottiglieri T, Laundy M, Crellin R, Toone BK, Carney MW, Reynolds EH: Homocysteine, folate, methylation, and monoamine metabolism in depression. J Neurol Neurosurg Psychiatry 2000; 69:228–232.

Alzheimer's disease could be considered a type of vascular disease, although it is much more complicated than a simple atherosclerotic build-up of plaque[150]. Cholesterol is implicated in the formation of the atherosclerotic plaques associated with Alzheimer's disease[151], but there is an additional mechanism that involves cholesterol in seeding the growth of the beta-amyloid peptides associated with the disease process[152]. However, there is a direct correlation between excessive cholesterol in the brain and Alzheimer's disease[153].

The dietary intervention to reduce and reverse vascular disease: whole-food varied-plant diet.

GENETICS

Certainly there is a genetic influence in the development of Alzheimer's disease but like so many other disorders thought to be inevitable based on genes, it appears to be just another risk

---

[150] Torre, J. C. (2002). Vascular Basis of Alzheimer's Pathogenesis. *Annals of the New York Academy of Sciences, 977*(1), 196-215. doi:10.1111/j.1749-6632.2002.tb04817.x.

[151] Corsinovi, L., Biasi, F., Poli, G., Leonarduzzi, G., & Isaia, G. (2011). Dietary lipids and their oxidized products in Alzheimer's disease. *Molecular Nutrition & Food Research Mol. Nutr. Food Res., 55*(S2). doi:10.1002/mnfr.201100208.

[152] Mizuno, T., Nakata, M., Naiki, H., Michikawa, M., Wang, R., Haass, C., & Yanagisawa, K. (1999). Cholesterol-dependent Generation of a Seeding Amyloid -Protein in Cell Culture. *Journal of Biological Chemistry, 274*(21), 15110-15114. doi:10.1074/jbc.274.21.15110.

[153] Reed, B., Villeneuve, S., Mack, W., Decarli, C., Chui, H. C., & Jagust, W. (2014). Associations Between Serum Cholesterol Levels and Cerebral Amyloidosis. *JAMA Neurology JAMA Neurol, 71*(2), 195. doi:10.1001/jamaneurol.2013.5390.

factor. And this genetic risk may be evolving to be less of a factor. Apolipoprotein E (ApoE) is a protein that is essential for the normal catabolism of triglyceride-rich lipoprotein constituents as found in meat. ApoE has a number of alternative forms that can result in different traits; the three forms are called ApoE2, ApoE3 and ApoE4. The ApoE4 variant, apparently predominant in pre-modern hominids, is a known genetic risk factor for impaired lipid

> *Dementia, including Alzheimer's disease is vascular in origin.*

regulation leading to elevated cholesterol, triglycerides and poor modulation of inflammation and oxidative stress, predisposing an individual to vascular disease and Alzheimer's disease.

However, this is less true of the ApoE3 (and ApoE2) variant that is dominant today (80%); the emergence of this increased frequency of the protective form of ApoE can be traced to within the past 200,000 years[154]. So it appears possible that as animal products have been introduced into the diet, there may have been a redistribution of the ApoE alleles in an attempt to partially offset disease processes.

EPIDEMIOLOGY

Because the molecular details of what causes Alzheimer's disease are unknown, we resort once again to epidemiologic studies.

---

[154] Fullerton, S., Clark, A., Weiss, K., Nickerson, D., Taylor, S., Stengård, J., . . . Sing, C. (2000). Apolipoprotein E Variation at the Sequence Haplotype Level: Implications for the Origin and Maintenance of a Major Human Polymorphism. *The American Journal of Human Genetics, 67*(4), 881-900.

The Mediterranean diet has been associated with a lower risk for Alzheimer's disease[155]. A review of a number of epidemiologic investigations on the effect of the Mediterranean diet on Alzheimer's disease indicated adherence to Mediterranean diet was able to affect not only the risk of incident disease but also the subsequent clinical course of the disease[156]. Adherence to the Mediterranean diet was linked to beneficial effects on some inflammatory and coagulation markers, lipids, and blood pressure, all important risk factors for Alzheimer's disease. An article in Science News titled "Dementia off the Menu" also indicated a Mediterranean-style diet was neuroprotective[157].

Another analysis of elderly subjects' dietary patterns followed over four years showed lower risk for developing Alzheimer's disease when there was higher intake of nuts, fish, tomatoes, poultry, cruciferous vegetables, fruits, and dark and green leafy vegetables, along with lower intake of high-fat diary products, red meat, organ meat, and butter [158] [159].

Comparisons between meat-eating and vegetarian subjects in Manhattan indicated a significantly higher incidence of

---

[155] Mohamed, H. E., El-Swefy, S. E., Rashed, L. A., & Abd El-Latif, S. K. (2010). Obesity and neurodegeneration: effect of a Mediterranean dietary pattern. *Nutritional Neuroscience, 13*(5), 205-212. doi:10.1179/147683010X12611460764444.

[156] Sofi, F., Macchi, C., Abbate, R., Gensini, G. F., & Casini, A. (2010). Effectiveness of the Mediterranean Diet: Can It Help Delay or Prevent Alzheimer's Disease? *Journal Of Alzheimer's Disease, 20*(3), 795-801. doi:10.3233/JAD-2010-1418.

[157] Harder, B. (2006). Dementia off the Menu. *Science News, 169*(16), 245.

[158] Abma, R. K. (2009). Nutrient Analysis Sheds New Light on Alzheimer's-Protective Diet. *Neurology Reviews, 17*(11), 18.

[159] Ferris, M. E. (2010). Dietary Choices with Lower Alzheimer's Disease Risk. *Internal Medicine Alert, 32*(18), 5.

Alzheimer's disease in the meat-eaters[160].　A prospective cohort study of over one thousand elderly Japanese implicated a linear relationship between the consumption of dairy products and Alzheimer's disease[161].

VASCULAR DISEASE CAUSES TISSUE DAMAGE

Damage to tissue results in an inflammatory response.　This is very protective to heal acute injuries, but when the inflammation is chronic and unhelpful, it can lead to problems in itself.　In the next chapter, we shall explore how chronic inflammation can lead to psychiatric disorders – and how to minimize them with dietary interventions.

AVOIDING SATURATED FAT

The liver uses saturated fat to make cholesterol, so eating foods with too much saturated fat can increase cholesterol levels, especially low-density lipoproteins (LDL)—the bad cholesterol. Saturated fats are usually found in animal products such as whole milk, cream, butter, and cheese, and meats such as beef, lamb and pork. There are some plant-based saturated fats you should avoid too, notably palm kernel oil, coconut oil, and vegetable shortening.

---

[160] Giem, P., Beeson, W. L., & Fraser, G. E. (1993). The Incidence of Dementia and Intake of Animal Products: Preliminary Findings from the Adventist Health Study. *Neuroepidemiology, 12*(1), 28-36. doi:10.1159/000110296.

[161] Ozawa, M., Ohara, T., Ninomiya, T., Hata, J., Yoshida, D., Mukai, N., & ... Kiyohara, Y. (2014). Milk and Dairy Consumption and Risk of Dementia in an Elderly Japanese Population: The Hisayama Study. *Journal Of The American Geriatrics Society, 62*(7), 1224-1230. doi:10.1111/jgs.12887.

CHAPTER 5

Neuroinflammation

"The best time to plant a tree is twenty years ago. The second best time is now."

Anonymous

PLANTS AS ANIMALS

Plants have an immune system that is nonspecific to each pathogen, quite similar to the animal "innate immune system"; there is no adaptive mechanism, no immunity through memory of specific pathogens. The innate immune system of plants is a necessity of their inability to move about evading invaders and a result of their extraordinary ability to manufacture defensive organic chemicals. Because of this powerful chemical production ability of plants, many hundreds of thousands of such compounds are made for protection from the large spectrum of potential attackers. Some act as simple toxins, others in much more complex ways.

Members of every class of pathogen which infect humans also infect plants. Similarities between the innate immune systems of plants and those of animals are considered "convergent evolution" and a consequence of inherent constraints on how such an innate immune system can be constructed[162]. That means that while there were some early common denominators of immune activity before eukaryotes diversified into the plant and animal kingdoms, most all of which we identify with immune defense in plant and animals have evolved separately, in parallel, but have similar properties.

These plant versus animal innate immune system stories have similar plots but completely different characters. One "plot twist" in the plant immune system story involves the use of pattern-recognition receptors to recognize microbes, utilizing a large number of manufactured "resistance" proteins. Those proteins are indeed a vast cast.

Unfortunately, the various immunity players in plants, while they do have analogs in animals, do not appear to be directly useful to humans in our immune systems when we eat them, although they may be. We just don't know yet[163].

ASPIRIN PLANT

Perhaps the first plant nutraceutic modified slightly to become a large commercial success was *salicylic acid*, found in particularly high amounts in the inner lining of white willow

---

[162] Ausubel FM., Are innate immune signaling pathways in plants and animals conserved?, Nat Immunol. 2005 Oct;6(10):973-9.

[163] "Consuming anti-microbial compounds (as well as other compounds) synthesized by plants as part of their immune response may be beneficial to human immunity. That is the only connection that I see between plant and human immunity", Ausubel, Frederick M, Department of Genetics, Harvard Medical School, Boston, Massachusetts private communication, July 2012.

tree bark and central to defense mechanisms in plants against pathogenic attack and environmental stress. It is the principal metabolite of the medication *aspirin*, which works through a completely different pathway in humans to affect an anti-inflammatory and antipyretic response. However, dosing in isolated concentrated form resulted in severe gastrointestinal distress, so a buffered form was developed – and patented – in 1900 as Aspirin (acetylsalicylic acid) by Bayer[164]. This approach to acquiring medicinal benefits from salicylic acid is still flawed by the fact that there is an increased risk of bleeding even with low-dose therapy. About one in ten people on chronic low-dose aspirin develop stomach or intestinal ulcers, which can perforate the gut and cause life-threatening bleeding.[165]

There is a better way to take advantage of the healing properties of salicylic acid: eating plants. All plants contain salicylic acid and some vegetarians have as much in their blood as omnivores who take aspirin supplements - but without the risk[166]. Apparently, this has been known empirically since the third millennium BC.

This is another recurring theme: varied - plant diets can obviate the need for many supplements and prescribed medications. Such diets are anti-inflammatory not only because of salicylic

---

[164] Interestingly, Aspirin ® and Heroin ® were once trademarks belonging to Bayer. After Germany lost World War I, Bayer was forced to give up both trademarks as part of the Treaty of Versailles in 1919.

[165] Yeomans, N., Lanas, A., Talley, N., Thomson, A., Daneshjoo, R., Eriksson, B., . . . Hawkey, C. (2005). Prevalence and incidence of gastroduodenal ulcers during treatment with vascular protective doses of aspirin. *Aliment Pharmacol Ther Alimentary Pharmacology and Therapeutics, 22*(9), 795-801.

[166] Paterson, J., Baxter, G., Dreyer, J., Halket, J., Flynn, R., & Lawrence, J. (2008). Salicylic Acid sans Aspirin in Animals and Man: Persistence in Fasting and Biosynthesis from Benzoic Acid. *Journal of Agricultural and Food Chemistry J. Agric. Food Chem., 56*(24), 11648-11652.

acid but because of their many other anti-inflammatory phytonutrients that help prevent the body from overproducing inflammatory compounds. Further, varied - plant diets minimize one's intake of inflammatory precursors present in meat and dairy products in the first place. More on that later.

Just to review, this amazing substance, salicylic acid, the active metabolite of aspirin and a plant hormone, plays a central role in the immune system of plants by activating the production of pathogen-fighting proteins[167]. It can transmit the distress signal throughout the plant and even to neighboring plants[168]. But the amazing fact is its crossover and apparent *inverse* role that it has in humans: it *reduces* the immune response, i.e. serves as an anti-inflammatory. This has an important role then in chronic inflammatory states such as cardio- and cerebrovascular disease, strokes, arthritis, even certain cancers. Recently, as mental disorders have been linked to chronic inflammatory states[169], aspirin is finding use for disorders ranging from mood disorders[170] to schizophrenia[171].

---

[167] Pieterse, C., Van Der Does, C., Zamioudis, C., Leon-Reyes, A., & Van Wees, S. (2012). *Hormonal modulation of plant immunity*. Annu Rev Cell Dev Biol.

[168] Taiz, L., & Zeiger, E. (2002). *Plant physiology* (3rd ed., p. 306). New York: W.H. Freeman.

[169] Berk, M., Dean, O., Drexhage, H., McNeil, J. J., Moylan, S., O'Neil, A., ... Maes, M. (2013). Aspirin a review of its neurobiological properties and therapeutic potential for mental illness. *BMC Medicine, 11*, 74. doi:10.1186/1741-7015-11-74.

[170] Ayorech, Z., Tracy, D., Baumeister, D., & Giaroli, G. (2015). Taking the fuel out of the fire: Evidence for the use of anti-inflammatory agents in the treatment of bipolar disorders. *Journal of Affective Disorders, 174*, 467-478.

[171] Keller, W., Kum, L., Wehring, H., Koola, M., Buchanan, R., & Kelly, D. (2012). A review of anti-inflammatory agents for symptoms of schizophrenia. *Journal of Psychopharmacology (Oxford, England), 27*(4), 337-342.

I IGNITE

First, let's be careful with our terms. *Inflammation* (from the Latin, *īnflammō*, "I ignite") is part of the complex biological response of tissues to perceived harmful stimuli, such as pathogens, damaged cells, or irritants. Inflammation is therefore intended to be part of the healing process. For example, an organism may be infected by an unwanted microorganism and inflammation is one of the responses of the organism to that pathogen.

It is remarkable to think that apart from accidents and suicide, humans primarily die from inadequate workings of the immune system (although even suicide, if not drug related or a permanent impulsive response to a temporary situation, may be related to an inflammatory process, as we shall see). On the one hand, we die of acute infections from the inadequate immune response to invading agents; this is the main cause of death in third-world countries. On the other hand, we also die from complications of a prolonged or chronic inflammation that might be thought of as an overactive innate immune response; this is the main cause of death in the Western world and includes vascular disease and cancer. The prevalence of chronic, degenerative diseases attributable wholly or in part to dietary patterns may be the most serious threat to public health in the United States[172].

There is now evidence that neuroinflammatory processes, that is, inflammation taking place in neural tissue, play an important role in depression in conjunction with enhanced neurodegeneration. Multiple inflammatory cytokines, oxygen radical damage, and neurodegenerative biomarkers have been established in patients with depression. Therefore, anti-

---

[172] Neustadt, J. (2011). Western diet and inflammation. *Integrative Medicine*.

inflammatory and anti-oxidative treatment, as present in select varied - plant diets, could be effective in alleviating depression.

Clinical depression, therefore, appears to be associated in part with the innate immune response as reflected by the increased biomarkers of inflammation[173]. Note that the innate immune response is different from the acquired or adaptive immune response which develops more slowly toward highly specific pathogens (called antigens) and produces antibodies with a memory of the antigen for future efficient response. Instead, the innate immune system provides a rapid, front-line defense against a variety of pathogens, toxins, and damaged cells, then recruits and activates various immune cells, leading to the typical clinical characteristics of inflammation.

These characteristics include weakness, fatigue, loss of energy and "the blahs", also known as "sickness behavior"[174]. Sickness behavior is related but differs from clinical depression; whereas acute infections typically elicit sickness behavior, there is not much evidence that acute response to pathogens plays a major role in clinical depression[175].

However, there is a high rate of depression in those with chronic inflammatory states. This includes people who are

---

[173] Including biomarkers of immune cytokines, acute-phase proteins, chemokines, and adhesion molecules; Raison CL, Capuron L, Miller AH: Cytokines sing the blues: inflammation and the pathogenesis of major depression. Trend Immunol 2006; 27:24–31.

[174] Also includes malaise, hyperalgesia, pyrexia, disinterest in social interactions, lethargy, behavioral inhibition, reduction of locomotor activity, reduction of reproductive performance, anhedonia, somnolence, anorexia and weight loss, failure to concentrate and anxiety.

[175] Maes, M., Berk, M., Goehler, L., Song, C., Anderson, G., Gałecki, P., & Leonard, B. (2012). Depression and sickness behavior are Janus-faced responses to shared inflammatory pathways. *BMC Medicine BMC Med, 10*(1), 66. doi:10.1186/1741-7015-10-66.

medically ill with disorders involving the immune system such as infectious diseases, cancer, and autoimmune disorders[176]; there is as much as a ten-fold increase in rates of clinical depression[177]. As the inflammatory response increases, so does the severity of depression[178]. Inflammation may not only act as a precipitating factor for depression but also as a perpetuating factor that may pose an obstacle to recovery.

Furthermore, there is an increasing understanding of the role that inflammation plays in vascular disease, and that fact provides yet another link to association with depression as described in the previous chapter[179].

Activation of the innate immune response has been linked to a number of pathophysiologic processes related to depression,

---

[176] Evans DL, Charney DS, Lewis L, Golden RN, Gorman JM, Krishnan KR, Nemeroff CB, Bremner JD, Carney RM, Coyne JC, Delong MR, Frasure-Smith N, Glassman AH, Gold PW, Grant I, Gwyther L, Ironson G, Johnson RL, Kanner AM, Katon WJ, Kaufmann PG, Keefe FJ, Ketter T, Laughren TP, Leserman J, Lyketsos CG, McDonald WM, McEwen BS, Miller AH, Musselman DL, O'Connor C, Petitto JM, Pollock BG, Robinson RG, Roose SP, Rowland J, Sheline Y, Sheps DS, Simon G, Spiegel D, Stunkard A, Sunderland T, Tibbits PJ, Valvo WJ: Mood disorders in the medically ill: scientific review and recommendations. Biol Psychiatry 2005; 58:175–189.

[177] Evans DL, Staab JP, Petitto JM, Morrison MF, Szuba MP, Ward HE, Wingate B, Luber MP, O'Reardon JP: Depression in the medical setting: biopsychological interactions and treatment considerations. J Clin Psychiatry 1999; 60(Suppl 4):40–55; discussion 56.

[178] Alan J. Thomas, I. Nicol Ferrier, Rajesh N. Kalaria, Susan A. Woodward, Clive Ballard, Arthur Oakley, Robert H. Perry, and John T. O'Brien, Elevation in Late-Life Depression of Intercellular Adhesion Molecule-1 Expression in the Dorsolateral Prefrontal Cortex, Am J Psychiatry, Oct 2000; 157: 1682 - 1684.

[179] Willerson JT, Ridker PM: Inflammation as a cardiovascular risk factor. Circulation 2004; 109:II2–II10.

including neurotransmitter metabolism leading to a decrease in serotonin, norepinephrine, and dopamine[180].

EPIDEMIOLOGIC EVIDENCE RELATING DIET TO INFLAMMATION

We have seen in Chapter 3 that epidemiologic data suggests a relationship between certain dietary patterns and adverse mood states. Can we break that association down further? What dietary patterns are associated with chronic inflammation and does the existence of chronic inflammatory states correlate with depression? These associations are not necessarily causative but, minimally, are useful in understanding risk factors.

Epidemiological data as well as human intervention studies suggest that dietary patterns emphasizing fruits and vegetables are strongly inversely proportional to inflammatory processes[181].

> *Consumption of plants is anti-inflammatory.*

A traditional Mediterranean dietary pattern, which typically has a higher ratio of monounsaturated to saturated fats, contains an abundance of fruits, vegetables, legumes, and grains, has shown anti-inflammatory effects when compared with typical North American and Northern European dietary patterns in

---

[180] Andrew H. Miller and Charles L. Raison, Immune System Contributions to the Pathophysiology of Depression, Focus, Winter 2008; 6: 36 - 45.

[181] Watzl, B. (2008). Anti-inflammatory Effects of Plant-based Foods and of their Constituents. *International Journal for Vitamin and Nutrition Research, 78*(6), 293-298.

most observational and interventional studies[182]. The Mediterranean dietary pattern may best fulfill requirements for an anti-inflammatory diet, at least when compared with other dietary patterns of the Western world.

However, inclusion of some foods that are not considered central to the Mediterranean diet would enhance its anti-inflammatory benefits, especially increased dark leafy greens, nuts such as walnuts, and seeds such as flax[183]. This is in part a result of the presence of omega-3 fatty acids; a diet disproportionately high in omega-6 fatty acids, which are commonly used in the production of processed foods, increases the production of pro-inflammatory cytokines[184].

Fiber, such as contained in whole grain foods, appears to have immune modulating functions. Fiber favorably influences gut microbiota[185], and this has a beneficial effect on immune functioning. Whole grain foods are also high in antioxidants, which protect against the oxidative stress that is a consequence of inflammation and a feature of depressive illness[186].

---

[182] Sofi, F., Fabbri, A., & Casini, A. (2016). Inflammation and Cardio-vascular Disease and Protection by the Mediterranean Diet. *Mediterranean Diet,* 89-96. doi:10.1007/978-3-319-27969-5_7.

[183] Galand, L. (2010). Diet and inflammation. Nutrition in clinical practice 25(6), 634-40.

[184] Rangel-Huerta, O. D., Aguilera, C. M., Mesa, M. D., & Gil, A. (2012). Omega-3 long-chain polyunsaturated fatty acids supplementation on inflammatory biomakers: A systematic review of randomised clinical trials. *British Journal of Nutrition Br J Nutr, 107*(S2). doi:10.1017/s0007114512001559.

[185] Tachon, S., Zhou, J., Keenan, M., Martin, R., & Marco, M. L. (2012). The intestinal microbiota in aged mice is modulated by dietary resistant starch and correlated with improvements in host responses. *FEMS Microbiol Ecol FEMS Microbiology Ecology, 83*(2), 299-309. doi:10.1111/j.1574-6941.2012.01475.x.

[186] Bilici, M., Efe, H., Köroğlu, M., Uydu, H. A., Bekaroğlu, M., & Değer, O. (2001). Antioxidative enzyme activities and lipid peroxidation in major

A review of the epidemiologic literature summarizing evidence on associations between dietary patterns and biomarkers of inflammation concluded[187]:

> *"Biomarkers of inflammation were almost all meat-based or 'Western' patterns. Studies using principal component analysis or a priori-defined diet scores found that meat-based or 'Western-like' patterns tended to be positively associated with biomarkers of inflammation, predominantly C-reactive protein, while vegetable- and fruit-based or 'healthy' patterns tended to be inversely associated with presumed ... healthy diets resulted in reductions of almost all investigated inflammatory biomarkers."*

Example anti-inflammatory bioactive phytonutritive compounds in plants include carotenoids and flavonoids. There are over 600 known carotenoids having a variety of colors ranging from pale yellow through bright orange to deep red. They serve two key roles in plants: they absorb light energy for use in photosynthesis, and they protect chlorophyll from photodamage[188]. There is an analogous function in humans as antioxidants in addition to their role in anti-inflammation.

---

depression: Alterations by antidepressant treatments. *Journal of Affective Disorders, 64*(1), 43-51. doi:10.1016/s0165-0327(00)00199-3.

[187] Barbaresko, J., Koch, M., Schulze, M. B., & Nöthlings, U. (2013). Dietary pattern analysis and biomarkers of low-grade inflammation: a systematic literature review. *Nutrition Reviews, 71*(8), 511-527. doi:10.1111/nure.12035.

[188] Armstrong, G., & Hearst, J. (1996). Carotenoids 2: Genetics and molecular biology of carotenoid pigment biosynthesis. *FASEB J, 10*(2), 228-237.

Flavonoids are also present in a wide variety of plants[189]. They serve many functions from ultraviolet filtration to floral pigmentation to attract pollinator animals. Generally they are plant hormones or chemical messengers that serve signaling functions, most of which are currently unknown to science. At one time, flavonoids were proposed as a class of vitamins, Vitamin P, but this was not generally adopted.

While plants are anti-inflammatory, what about animal products? We know that a single meal high in animal fat can cause an elevation in inflammation within our bodies that peaks at about four hours[190]. After a meal of animal products, we develop *endotoxemia*, a condition in which our bloodstream contains bacterial toxins, known as *endotoxins*. So inflammation is produced from endotoxins in the bacteria from animal products.

Dietary patterns including animals and animal products contribute to chronic inflammation that is associated with neuropsychiatric disease.

So it's the bacteria present in *meat products and processed foods* that bring the endotoxins[191]. And it doesn't matter if the bacteria is dead or alive – even subjected to high temperatures (as in cooking) or highly acidic environments (as in our stomachs), because it is the biochemical bacteria-derived

---

[189] Spencer, J. (2008). Flavonoids: Modulators of brain function? *BJN British Journal of Nutrition, 99,* 60-77.

[190] Vogel, R., Corretti, M., & Plotnick, G. (1997). Effect of a Single High-Fat Meal on Endothelial Function in Healthy Subjects. *The American Journal of Cardiology, 79*(3), 350-354.

[191] Erridge, C. (2010). The capacity of foodstuffs to induce innate immune activation of human monocytes in vitro is dependent on food content of stimulants of Toll-like receptors 2 and 4. *Br J Nutr British Journal of Nutrition, 105*(1), 15-23.

endotoxins not the bacteria itself that causes the damage. Saturated fat, also present in animal products, has an important role in assisting the endotoxin transport through the gastrointestinal endothelium.

Plants boost immune function in humans but do not trigger the immune response. Animal products do.

ASSOCIATION OF INFLAMMATION WITH DEPRESSION

We have seen in Chapter 4 that there is an apparent correlation between certain dietary patterns and positive or negative mood states. In the last section, we saw that diet can be correlated with chronic inflammatory states. To close the loop, in this section we shall explore the correlation of inflammation to adverse mood states.

Most of the evidence that links inflammation to depressed mood states comes from three observations[192]:

- One-third of those with depression show elevated peripheral inflammatory biomarkers, even in the absence of a medical illness.
- Inflammatory illnesses are associated with greater rates of depression.
- Patients treated with cytokines, creating an inflammatory state, are at greater risk of developing major depressive illness.

To illustrate this last point, it is noted that a high percentage of patients who are administered the cytokine interferon for the

---

[192] Krishnadas, R., & Cavanagh, J. (2012). Depression: An inflammatory illness?: Figure 1. *Journal of Neurology, Neurosurgery & Psychiatry J Neurol Neurosurg Psychiatry, 83*(5), 495-502. doi:10.1136/jnnp-2011-301779.

treatment of infectious diseases or cancer develop an emotional, behavioral syndrome that is strikingly similar - if not identical - to clinical depression[193].

We have explored the effect of diet on the emergence of chronic inflammatory states but other factors can exacerbate the condition including psychosocial stressors, physical inactivity, obesity, smoking, altered gut permeability, dental cares, insufficient sleep, and vitamin D deficiency[194]. Most of these factors are amenable to preventative and restorative life-style interventions. These sources of inflammation may play a role not only in the development of clinical depression but possibly have an influence on the etiology of other psychiatric disorders, such as bipolar disorder, schizophrenia, autism and post-traumatic stress disorder[195] [196].

It has been postulated that the impact of inflammation on behavior is associated not exclusively with depression but with specific symptom dimensions across diagnoses that align with the Research Domain Criteria framework put forth by the

---

[193] Capuron, L., & Miller, A. H. (2004). Cytokines and psychopatholo-gy: Lessons from interferon-α. *Biological Psychiatry, 56*(11), 819-824. doi:10.1016/j.biopsych.2004.02.009.

[194] Berk, M., Williams, L. J., Jacka, F. N., O'Neil, A., Pasco, J. A., Moy-lan, S., . . . Maes, M. (2013). So depression is an inflammatory disease, but where does the inflammation come from? *BMC Medicine BMC Med, 11*(1). doi:10.1186/1741-7015-11-200.

[195] Maes, M., Bosmans, E., Calabrese, J., Smith, R., & Meltzer, H. Y. (1995). Interleukin-2 and interleukin-6 in schizophrenia and mania: Ef-fects of neuroleptics and mood stabilizers. *Journal of Psychiatric Re-search, 29*(2), 141-152. doi:10.1016/0022-3956(94)00049-w.

[196] Modabbernia, A., Taslimi, S., Brietzke, E., & Ashrafi, M. (2013). Cy-tokine Alterations in Bipolar Disorder: A Meta-Analysis of 30 Stud-ies. *Biological Psychiatry, 74*(1), 15-25. doi:10.1016/ j.biopsych. 2013.01.007.

National Institute of Mental Health[197]. These symptoms relate to decreased motivation and motor activity, anhedonia, fatigue and increased anxiety, arousal and alarm[198].

DIETARY INTERVENTIONS FOR INFLAMMATORY-RELATED DEPRESSIVE DISORDERS

The use of conventional antidepressants has been a notable achievement in psychiatry since the mid-twentieth century. Unfortunately, a significant fraction – perhaps as high as two-thirds - of mild to moderate clinically depressed individuals do not achieve full remission as a result of the use of an antidepressant alone[199].

Given that there does appear to be a strong association of clinical depression with chronic inflammation, it is natural to consider attenuating inflammatory-mediated processes as a supplementary treatment[200]. Studies have found that certain

---

[197] Morris, S. E. & Cuthbert, B. N. (2012) Research Domain Criteria: cognitive systems, neural circuits, and dimensions of behavior. Dialogues Clin. Neurosci. 14, 29–37.

[198] Miller, A. H., & Raison, C. L. (2015). The role of inflammation in depression: From evolutionary imperative to modern treatment target. *Nat Rev Immunol Nature Reviews Immunology, 16*(1), 22-34. doi:10.1038/nri.2015.5.

[199] Rush J, Trivedi M, Wisniewski S, Nierenberg A, Stewart J, Warden D, Niederehe G, Thase M, Lavori P, Lebowitz B, Mcgrath P, Rosenbaum J, Sackeim H, Kupfer D, Luther J, Fava M (2006) Acute and longer-term outcomes in depressed outpatients requiring one or several: a STAR*D report. Am J Psychiatry 163:1905–1917.

[200] Fond G, Hamdani N, Kapczinski F, Boukouaci W, Drancourt N, Dargel A, Oliveira J, Le Guen E, Marlinge E, Tamouza R, Leboyer M (2014) Effectiveness and tolerance of anti- inflammatory drugs' add-on therapy in major mental disorders: a systematic qualitative review. Acta Psychiatr Scand 129:163–179.

inflammatory cytokines predict poor response to conventional antidepressant therapy[201].

PUFAs

Polyunsaturated fatty acids (PUFAs) are omega-3 fatty acids derived entirely from dietary plant and marine sources, and include alpha linolenic acid (ALA), eicosapentaenoic (EPA) and docosahexaenoic acid (DHA). Their main function is to act as an essential component of membranes, such as those of neurons, and also to give rise to eicosanoids, which affect inflammation[202]. Eicosanoids from omega-3 fatty acids reduce the synthesis of arachidonic acid-derived eicosanoids that are pro-inflammatory, and it is the balance between these fatty acids which maintains an equilibrium in the immune system.

Flaxseed, hemp, canola and walnuts are all generally rich sources of the parent omega-3, ALA. Dietary ALA can be metabolized in the liver to the longer-chain omega-3 EPA and DHA. It is estimated that only 5–15% of ALA is ultimately converted to DHA[203]. Aging, illness and stress, as well as excessive amounts of omega-6 rich oils (corn, safflower, sunflower, cottonseed) can all compromise conversion[204].

---

[201] Cattaneo A, Gennarelli M, Uher R, Breen G, Farmer A, Aitchison KJ, Craig IW, Anacker C, Zunsztain PA, Mcguffin P, Pariante CM (2013) Candidate genes expression profile associated with antidepressants response in the GENDEP study: differentiating between baseline 'predictors' and longitudinal 'targets'. Neuropsychopharmacology 38:377–385.

[202] Das UN (2006) Essential fatty acids: biochemistry, physiology and pathology. Biotechnol J 1:420–439.

[203] Holub BJ: Clinical nutrition: 4. Omega-3 fatty acids in cardio- vascular care. CMAJ 2002, 166:608-615.

[204] Bourre, J. M. (2009). Diet, Brain Lipids, and Brain Functions: Polyunsaturated Fatty Acids, Mainly Omega-3 Fatty Acids. *Handbook of Neurochemistry and Molecular Neurobiology,* 409-441. doi:10.1007/978-0-387-30378-9_17.

Dietary fish and seafood provide varying amounts of pre-formed EPA and DHA.

Consumption of omega-6 PUFAs increases the production of pro-inflammatory cytokines and consumption of omega-3 PUFAs reduces the activity of these omega-6 PUFAs, therefore reducing inflammation. The therapeutic use of omega-3 PUFAs for inflammatory conditions has long been known.

We evolved genetic patterns established on a diet with a ratio of omega-6 to omega-3 essential fatty acids (EFA) of approximately 1, whereas in Western diets the ratio is about 16. This high ratio promotes the pathogenesis of vascular disease, cancer, and inflammatory and autoimmune diseases, whereas lower ratios exert suppressive effects[205].

A distorted ratio of these polyunsaturated fatty acids may be one of the most damaging aspects of the Western diet, leading to chronic inflammation and resulting vascular diseases and adverse mood states[206].

The plot below illustrates the ratio of omega-3 to omega-6 for select foods.

---

[205] Simopoulos, A. (2002). The importance of the ratio of omega-6/omega-3 essential fatty acids. *Biomedicine & Pharmacotherapy, 56*(8), 365-379.

[206] Simopoulos AP (2008) The importance of the omega-6/omega-3 fatty acid ratio in cardio-vascular disease and other chronic diseases. Exp Biol Med (Maywood) 233:674–688.

Figure 4 Omega-3 to Omega-6 Ratio

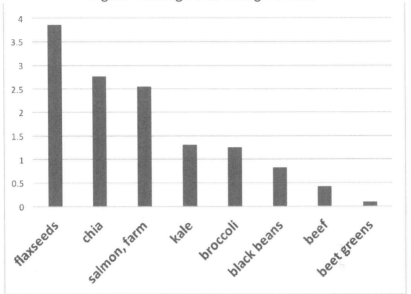

Typical cruciferous vegetables (cauliflower, cabbage, bok choy, broccoli, Brussel sprouts and similar green vegetables) contain the ratio experienced by our primate ancestors. Legumes are acceptable sources for these essential fats as well. Flaxseeds have an extraordinarily favorable content of these nutrients and can be used in small quantities to assure adequate intake.

Epidemiological evidence suggests that dietary omega-3 PUFAs reduce the risk of clinical depression, seasonal affective disorder, bipolar disorder and post-partum depression[207]. This has been demonstrated in the Mediterranean diet, where there is a decreased prevalence and incidence of depression, with the consumption of oily fish is presumably the dietary source of

---

[207] Mcnamara RK (2015) Mitigation of inflammation-induced mood dysregulation by long-chain omega-3 fatty acids. J Am Coll Nutr 34(Suppl 1):48–55.

omega-3 PUFAs[208]. There are many other healthy aspects of the Mediterranean diet, so it is not possible to point toward a single component of the diet as being the primary healthy element.

This correlation has also been supported in parts of Asia, for example Japan and Korea, where the diet is higher in omega-3 rich seafood. One study found that, in a sample of 500 Japanese participants, increased fish consumption was associated with resilience to depression[209]. Another study with Korean participants and controls, demonstrated that the increased consumption of seafood was associated with a decreased risk of depression[210].

Omega-3 PUFAs have been shown to be successful when used as an adjunctive therapy to antidepressants[211]. A double-blind placebo-controlled trial compared 9.6 g/ day of PUFAs or placebo in addition to usual treatment of an antidepressant

> *Omega-3 fatty acids are antiinflammatory and do have a positive correlation with cognitive and emotional health. An excellent single source of omega-3s is flax seeds.*

---

[208] Rienks J, Dobson AJ, Mishra GD (2013) Mediterranean dietary pattern and prevalence and incidence of depressive symptoms in mid-aged women: results from a large community-based prospective study. Eur J Clin Nutr 67:75–82.

[209] Yoshikawa E, Nishi D, Matsuoka Y (2015) Fish consumption and resilience to depression in Japanese company workers: a cross-sectional study. Lipids Health Dis 14:51.

[210] Park Y, Kim M, Baek D, Kim S (2012) Erythrocyte n-3 polyunsaturated fatty acid and seafood intake decrease the risk of depression: case-control study in Korea. Ann Nutr Metab 61:25–31.

[211] Stoll AL, Severus WE, Freeman MP, Rueter S, Zboyan HA, Diamond E, Cress KK, Marangell LB (1999) Omega 3 fatty acids in bipolar disorder: a preliminary double-blind, placebo-controlled trial. Arch Gen Psychiatry 56:407–412.

for four months; the group receiving omega-3 PUFAs had a longer remission rate and performed better on the majority of outcome measures when compared to the placebo group. In another study[212], 2 grams of EPA were added to antidepressant medication for patients with clinical depression, and results implied that omega-3 PUFAs may boost the antidepressant effects of traditional medication. Note that the EPAs used in these studies were ethyl eicosapentaenoic acid (E-EPA) from *purified* fish oil.

Omega-3 PUFAs have also been used alone without antidepressants to good effect in a small pilot study that examined 20 children between the ages of 6–12, who had suffered from depression for an average of 3 months. The placebo-controlled prospective trial gave the treatment cohort 400 mg of EPA and 200 mg of DHA daily, and 7 out of 10 children had a greater than 50% reduction in the Children's Depression Rating Scale when compared to 0 out of 10 children achieving this in the placebo group[213].

However, the success of these supplements seems to be associated with the level of EPA, rather than DHA[214] [215]; note

---

[212] Nemets B, Stahl Z, Belmaker RH (2002) Addition of omega-3 fatty acid to maintenance medication treatment for recurrent unipolar depressive disorder. Am J Psychiatry 159:477–479.

[213] Nemets H, Nemets B, Apter A, Bracha Z, Belmaker RH (2006) Omega-3 treatment of childhood depression: a controlled, double-blind pilot study. Am J Psychiatry 163:1098–1100.

[214] Grosso G, Pajak A, Marventano S, Castellano S, Galvano F, Bucolo C, Drago F, Caraci F (2014) Role of omega-3 fatty acids in the treatment of depressive disorders: a comprehensive meta-analysis of randomized clinical trials. PLoS One 9, e96905.

[215] Song C, Shieh C, Wu Y, Kalueff A, Gaikwad S, Su K (2016) The role of omega-3 polyunsaturated fatty acids eicosapentaenoic and docosahexaenoic acids in the treatment of major depression and Alz-

there is some inconsistency in other similar research and the degree of deficiency of omega-3s prior to the studies may have had an influence.

PUFA SOURCES

Theoretically it appears that a diet with significant fish consumption should satisfy our need for omega-3 PUFAs through the preformed EPA and DHA. Not so fast. Our oceans are so polluted that a variety of toxic persistent organic pollutants, such as dioxins, pesticides, polychlorinated biphenyls (PCBs), as well as heavy metals such as mercury, lead, and cadmium, may be present and adversely affect our health[216].

The emerging evidence suggests that omega-3 PUFAs from most commercially available fatty fish have no significant benefits on vascular disease[217]. This is likely a result of the exposure of fish to a wide variety of chemical contaminants and of altered fish dietary compositions due to commercial farming practices.

The research studies quoted above utilize carefully purified sources of EPA and DHA; results will vary considerably depending upon the dietary fish source.

---

heimer's disease: acting separately or synergistically? Prog Lipid Res 4:41–54.

[216] Jacobs, D. R., Ruzzin, J., & Lee, D. (2014). Environmental pollutants: Downgrading the fish food stock affects chronic disease risk. *J Intern Med Journal of Internal Medicine, 276*(3), 240-242. doi:10.1111/joim.12205.

[217] Kromhout D, Yasuda S, Geleijnse JM, et al. (2011) Fish oil and omega-3 fatty acids in cardiovascular disease: do they really work? Eur Heart J 33, 436–443.

Nuts

Nuts are nutrient-dense, rich in PUFAs such as ALA, high-quality plant protein, fiber, minerals, vitamins, and other bioactive compounds such as phytosterols and antioxidants[218].

One analysis of cross-sectional data from 5013 participants in the Nurses' Health Study and Health Professionals Follow-Up Study showed that a greater intake of nuts was associated with lower levels of a set of inflammatory biomarkers, after adjusting for demographic, medical, dietary, and lifestyle variables[219]. The researchers conclude:

> *"Substituting nuts for red and processed meat, eggs, refined grains, potatoes, or potato chips was associated with a healthier profile of inflammatory markers. These data support an overall healthful role of nuts in the diet and suggest an inverse association with inflammation."*

In that study, "nuts" included all sources including peanuts, tree nuts, and peanut butter.

ARACHIDONIC ACID

There is another substance analogous to cholesterol that we need and make in our own bodies, as do all animals, but do not

---

[218] Brufau, G., Boatella, J., & Rafecas, M. (2006). Nuts: Source of energy and macronutrients. *BJN British Journal of Nutrition, 96*(S2). doi:10.1017/bjn20061860.

[219] Yu, Z., Malik, V. S., Keum, N., Hu, F. B., Giovannucci, E. L., Stampfer, M. J., . . . Bao, Y. (2016). Associations between nut consumption and inflammatory biomarkers. *American Journal of Clinical Nutrition*. doi:10.3945/ajcn.116.134205.

want contributions of it from animals that we consume: namely, the omega-6 arachidonic acid (AA) mentioned earier. AA is a key substrate for the synthesis of proinflammatory compounds that can adversely affect mental health via a cascade of neuroinflammation[220].

Diets rich in meat and poultry are high in neuroinflammatory AA[221]. A randomized controlled study of omnivores with a significant EPA and DHA intake, but high AA/EPA and AA/DHA ratios showed a marked improvement in mood when shifted to a vegetarian diet with negligible EPA and DHA intake but also negligible AA[222].

STRESS AND INFLAMMATION

Chronic stress, from physiologic or psychologic triggers, has been associated with increased release of proinflammatory cytokines and decreases in anti-inflammatory cytokines[223]. The activation of the innate immune responses following stress and during depression might come at the expense of the acquired

---

[220] Beezhold, B., Johnston, C., & Daigle, D. (2010). Vegetarian diets are associated with healthy mood states: A cross-sectional study in Seventh Day Adventist adults. *Nutr J Nutrition Journal, 9,* 26-26.

[221] Farooqui, A. A., Horrocks, L. A., & Farooqui, T. (2006). Modulation of inflammation in brain: A matter of fat. *Journal of Neurochemistry, 101*(3), 577-599. doi:10.1111/j.1471-4159.2006.04371.x.

[222] Beezhold, B. L., & Johnston, C. S. (2012). Restriction of meat, fish, and poultry in omnivores improves mood: A pilot randomized controlled trial. *Nutrition Journal Nutr J, 11*(1). doi:10.1186/1475-2891-11-9.

[223] Goebel, M. U., Mills, P. J., Irwin, M. R., & Ziegler, M. G. (2000). Interleukin-6 and Tumor Necrosis Factor-α Production After Acute Psychological Stress, Exercise, and Infused Isoproterenol: Differential Effects and Pathways. *Psychosomatic Medicine, 62*(4), 591-598. doi:10.1097/00006842-200007000-00019.

immune responses, resulting in increased susceptibility to infections[224].

An important point here is that not only does tissue damage and infection lead to an innate immune response but so does other environmental stressors such as psychosocial stress[225] [226]. The social stress need not be extreme and prolonged and lead to clinical depression; one study merely required normal subjects to perform speaking and arithmetic tasks in front of an audience[227].

So while stress can precipitate inflammatory responses, inflammation can trigger oxidative stress. Clinical depression is accompanied by increased oxidative stress[228]. We shall investigate oxidative stress in the next chapter.

---

[224] Raison, C. L., & Miller, A. H. (2003). When Not Enough Is Too Much: The Role of Insufficient Glucocorticoid Signaling in the Pathophysiology of Stress-Related Disorders. *American Journal of Psychiatry AJP, 160*(9), 1554-1565. doi:10.1176/appi.ajp.160.9.1554.

[225] Pace, T. W., Mletzko, T. C., Alagbe, O., Musselman, D. L., Nemeroff, C. B., Miller, A. H., & Heim, C. M. (2006). Increased Stress-Induced Inflammatory Responses in Male Patients With Major Depression and Increased Early Life Stress. American Journal of Psychiatry AJP, 163(9), 1630-1633. doi:10.1176/ajp.2006.163.9.1630.

[226] Interleukin-1 beta: A putative mediator of HPA axis hyperactivity in major depression? (1993). American Journal of Psychiatry, 150(8), 1189-1193. doi:10.1176/ajp.150.8.1189.

[227] Bierhaus, A., Wolf, J., Andrassy, M., Rohleder, N., Humpert, P. M., Petrov, D., . . . Nawroth, P. P. (2003). A mechanism converting psychosocial stress into mononuclear cell activation. Proceedings of the National Academy of Sciences, 100(4), 1920-1925. doi:10.1073/pnas.0438019100.

[228] Leonard, B., & Maes, M. (2012). Mechanistic explanations how cell-mediated immune activation, inflammation and oxidative and nitrosative stress pathways and their sequels and concomitants play a role in the pathophysiology of unipolar depression. *Neuroscience & Biobehavioral Reviews, 36*(2), 764-785. doi:10.1016/j.neubiorev.2011.12.005.

CHAPTER 6

Stress

"The less effort, the faster and more powerful you will be. "

Bruce Lee

INTRODUCTION

Stress is a reaction to a stimulus that threatens our physical or mental equilibrium. If there is insufficient stasis or if the stress is chronic, this positive adaptive mechanism can become a negative intrusion and quite damaging in a number of ways.

Chronic inflammation, the topic of the last chapter, and stress are intimately related in a bi-directional way: either one can cause or amplify the other.

THE SUBCELLULAR ORIGIN OF OXIDATIVE STRESS

On the one hand, the simple prokaryotic bacterium *Rickettsia prowazekii*, or *Typhus*, is responsible for precipitating some of the worst plagues ever to afflict the human race. On the other hand, recent genome sequencing[229] has revealed that its evolutionary antecedent participated in one of the seminal events in the evolution of life as we know it. After it was "eaten" or otherwise introduced into the eukaryotic cell[230], the engulfed bacterium was able to keep much of its chemical composition and exist as a distinct entity inside the larger cell. This was a testament to the virulence of this particular bacterial strain. A new kind of mutual advantage occurred in this coexistence.

The new intracellular modified Typhus bacterium became known as the mitochondrion, the "cellular power plant" generating most of the cell's supply of chemical energy. So the "eaten" bacterium now within the larger cell is "fed" chemical substrates in trade for overall increased cellular energy, and the predator-prey distinction is obscured by this symbiosis. A Frankensteinian combination of cellular parts was brought alive by chemical "lightning".

The chemical processes taking place within the mitochondrion involve carbohydrates reacting with oxygen to produce water, carbon dioxide, and energy. This energy, in the form of a currency known as *ATP*, drives the growth, reproduction, and maintenance of the cell. Collectively, the many reactions involved in this energy production are called *glycolysis,* and although carbohydrates are the main fuel, fats and proteins can also participate directly although less efficiently.

This aerobic respiration is why we breathe, obtaining oxygen, and why we eat, obtaining primarily carbohydrates and secondarily protein and fat as fuel for our engines.

---

[229] Gray, M.W. (1998). Rickettsia, typhus and the mitochondrial connection. *Nature. 396, 109-110.*

[230] This process is termed *endiocytosis.*

This can be a very dangerous business, though, because of intermediate energy carrying molecules, called *free radicals*. These free radicals aren't the peace loving, anti-war protester types - they can freely cause radical cellular damage contributing to disease and aging. This is termed *oxidative stress*. To the rescue come other intra-cellular characters called *antioxidants*. When the oxidative stress is greater than that which the cell can control, damage results. An exogenous source of antioxidants comes from another perhaps even *more* profound example of cellular survival of mutually beneficial organisms. This happened about a billion years ago, give or take a few hundred million years[231].

It also involved a bacterium that was taken up by a eukaryote - the *cyanobacterium*, also known as blue green algae. That structure evolved into the *chloroplast*, a cell within the eukaryotic cell which provides photosynthetic production of energy from sunlight[232]. Such single-cell eukaryotes evolved into multicellular precursors of present day plant life. Please refer to the following illustration.

---

[231] Mcfadden, G., & Dooren, G. (2004). Evolution: Red Algal Genome Affirms a Common Origin of All Plastids. *Current Biology, 14*(13).

[232] Recent electron micrographs have shown a glimpse at how scientists think early organisms acquired free-living chloroplasts, which helped raise oxygen levels in Earth's atmosphere and paved the way for the rise of animals. See Maruyama, S., & Kim, E. (2012). A Modern Descendant of Early Green Algal Phagotrophs. *Current Biology, 23*(12), 1081-1084.

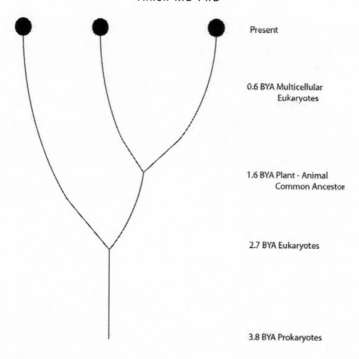

Present

0.6 BYA Multicellular Eukaryotes

1.6 BYA Plant - Animal Common Ancestor

2.7 BYA Eukaryotes

3.8 BYA Prokaryotes

Photosynthesis taking part in the eukaryotic cell marks the most recognized departure point in the evolution of plants versus animals, although the last common ancestor (LCA) was probably much before, at about 1.6 billion years ago[233]. In the process of photosynthesis, atmospheric carbon dioxide, together with water and sunlight, produces oxygen and carbohydrates. This complemented the glycolysis (outlined above); so the plants provide the fuel (carbohydrates) and the fire (oxygen) for animal life.

This sun-supercharged eukaryotic ancestor of plants, however, is quite independent of the precursor photosynthesis-less co-existing eukaryotes which took a different evolutionary track to become animals. Plant life proliferated and as a result, the oxygen composition of the atmosphere increased to a level that

---

[233] Meyerowitz, E. (2002). Plants Compared to Animals: The Broadest Comparative Study of Development. *Science, 295*(5559), 1482-1485.

encouraged the development of aerobic organisms such as animals.

TAMING THE FIRE — THE PURPOSE OF ANTIOXIDANTS

The defining moment in the divergence of plant from animal evolution was the adaptation leading to photosynthesis. The resulting chemical flame, or oxidative capacity, far exceeded that of simple glycolysis, the other energy production mechanism of plants and the only one for animals. The highly reactive — and potentially destructive - free radical chemical intermediates require antioxidants to control the process of glycolysis. This need for antioxidants is even greater during photosynthesis, where very highly reactive oxygen intermediates are produced[234].

As plants adapted to a terrestrial environment from marine life, they began producing non-marine antioxidants such as ascorbic acid[235] (vitamin C) and polyphenols. The evolution of flowering plants between 50 and 200 million years ago resulted in the development of many antioxidants in the form of pigments,

> *Oxidative stress is a natural result of subcellular energy production but must be balanced with antioxidants. Plants produce strong anti-oxidants that humans have evolved to rely upon.*

---

[234]Demmig-Adams, B. (2002). Antioxidants in Photosynthesis and Human Nutrition. *Science, 298*(5601), 2149-2153.
[235] Padayatty, S., Katz, A., Wang, Y., Eck, P., Kwon, O., Lee, J., . . . Levine, M. (2003). Vitamin C as an Antioxidant: Evaluation of Its Role in Disease Prevention. *Journal of the American College of Nutrition, 22*(1), 18-35.

compounds that reflect certain wavelengths of sunlight, appearing as various colors.[236] Absorption or reflection of sunlight, including that in the visible light spectrum, acts to control oxidative processes under conditions of high light intensity present on land compared to marine environments.

PHYSIOLOGIC OXIDATIVE STRESS

The development of various chronic and degenerative diseases, like cancer, vascular disease, and neuronal degeneration such as Alzheimer's and Parkinson's may be attributed, in part, to oxidative stress. Oxidative stress has also been implicated in the aging process. Although the human body has developed a number of systems to eliminate free radicals, it is not very efficient[237].

We therefore benefit from consuming plants, the champion antioxidant producers. Humans, for example, have apparently evolved with such a reliance on plants as the source of antioxidants that we no longer produce one of the most important antioxidants, vitamin C, present in all plants but essentially unavailable from animal food sources.

The primary fuel for our bodies is glucose, a simple sugar packed with energy. But you have likely heard of the perils of consuming products containing high levels of simple sugars, for example corn syrup. The problem lies in rapid and extensive oxidation of simple sugars that leads to the production of free radicals, a dangerous consequence as mentioned previously.

---

[236] Benzie, J. (2003). Evolution of dietary antioxidants. *Comparative Biochemistry and Physiology, 136*(1), 113-126.

[237] Seeram, N., Aviram, M., Zhang, Y., Henning, S., Feng, L., Dreher, M., & Heber, D. (2008). Comparison of Antioxidant Potency of Commonly Consumed Polyphenol-Rich Beverages in the United States. Journal of Agricultural and Food Chemistry J. Agric. Food Chem., 56, 1415-1422.

This might appear paradoxical, the most basic of fuels producing dangerous by-products.

The explanation is *synergy*. Consumption of extracts from foods, that is, not the whole food, can lead to problems. In the case of high sugar content foods, whole foods such as fruits are energy dense with sugars but also contain antioxidants. So although the sugars do lead to oxidation, there is no oxidative damage because of the accompanying antioxidants. Without sufficient intake of protective antioxidants, only found in plants, excessive intake of the typical energy-dense foods of Western societies can result in cellular dysfunction, disease, and death[238].

Dr. T. Colin Campbell, famed epidemiologist and co-author of *The China Study*[239] and more recently co-author of *Whole: Rethinking the Science of Nutrition*[240], remarks:

> *"Most importantly, however, we need to understand that these chemicals (nutrients) work in a highly integrated, virtually symphonic manner to produce their health effect. Thus it is a matter of thinking about the collection of such chemicals in large groups of foods. I hold that we need to discard the traditional view of nutrition, based on the effects of single nutrients, and take*

---

[238] Prior, R., Gu, L., Wu, X., Jacob, R., Sotoudeh, G., Kader, A., & Cook, R. (2007). Plasma Antioxidant Capacity Changes Following a Meal as a Measure of the Ability of a Food to Alter In Vivo Antioxidant Status. *Journal of the American College of Nutrition, 26*(2), 170-181.

[239] Campbell, T., & Campbell, T. (2005). *The China study: The most comprehensive study of nutrition ever conducted and the startling implications for diet, weight loss and long-term health.* Dallas, Tex.: BenBella Books.

[240] Campbell, T., & Jacobson, H. (2014). *Whole: Rethinking the Science of Nutrition.* BenBella Books.

seriously the symphonic nature of food chemicals working together. In effect, the 'whole' nutritional effect is greater than the sum of its parts[241]."

FOOD SYNERGY

Less than one half of one percent of all money for medical research is spent on whole food nutrition research, largely because there are no patented, profitable drugs that result[242]. Most research conducted takes the reductionist approach aimed at identifying the molecules involved in biological events and examining them in their purified form or in simple systems, often at much higher concentrations than appear in nature[243]. While this approach is understandable to isolate specific cause and effect, it misses the contextual aspect. Primarily epidemiologic studies of dietary patterns have been utilized, but this reduces the understanding of particular beneficial food combinations.

During the first half of the 20th century, a period often referred to as the Golden Age of Nutrition, all of the vitamins known today were identified, and good nutrition was viewed in terms of avoiding deficiency diseases - the reductionist perspective. This encouraged a collective vitamin pill supplementation.

---

[241] The Daily Beet. (n.d.). Retrieved May 27, 2015, from http://engine2diet.com/the-daily-beet/the-big-oil-post-plus-a-giveaway

[242] The Influence of Nutrition on Mental Health (Part 2) - Charis Holistic Center. (2011, October 26). Retrieved May 27, 2015, from http://www.charisholisticcenter.com/the-influence-of-nutrition-on-mental-health-part-2/.

[243] Zeisel, S., Allen, L., Coburn, S., Erdman, J., Failla, M., Freake, H., . . . Storch, J. (2001). Nutrition: A reservoir of integrative science. J Nutr, 131, 1319–1321-1319–1321.

Linus Pauling created the field of *Orthomolecular Nutrition*, "pertaining to the right molecule". Pauling proposed that by giving the body the right molecules in the right concentration, nutrients could be used by people to achieve better health and prolong life. He advocated the popular but controversial *megavitamin therapy* movement of the 1970s, particularly for vitamin C. This was a natural reductionist approach for a Nobel Prize winning molecular chemist (1954 in Chemistry for elucidating the nature of the chemical bond) but is widely considered to be a medical fail.

The concept of food synergy is based instead on the idea that the interrelations among constituents in foods are significant. But this is also true between foods, that is combinations of different whole foods.

Whole foods are greater than the sum of their individual constituents.

For example, the plant turmeric, containing the ingredient curcumin, appears to have a wide range of biological effects including anti-inflammatory, antioxidant, antibacterial, and antiviral[244], but is poorly absorbed, known as low *bioavailability*. With the addition of black pepper, and its active ingredient *piperine*, the bioavailability increases by 2000%.

The synergy likely works best with a variety of different fruits and vegetables. Extracts of phytonutrients, such as curcumin just mentioned, could have deleterious effects[245]. As

---

[244] Aggarwal, B., Sundaram, C., Malani, N., & Ichikawa, H. (2007). Curcumin: The Indian Solid Gold. The Molecular Targets and Therapeutic Uses of Curcumin in Health and Disease. Advances in Experiementa; Medicine and Biology, 595(1), 1-75.

[245] Cao, J., Jia, L., & Zhong, L. (2006). Mitochondrial and Nuclear DNA Damage Induced by Curcumin in Human Hepatoma G2 Cells. Toxicological Sciences, 91(2), 476-483.

phytonutrients have medicinal properties, it's probably best not to flood one's diet with only a few plant sources.

There are a number of known specific examples of food combinations that appear to have synergy. Fats make carotenoids more bioavailable, so a combination of tomatoes and avocados may be a good one. Tomatoes and broccoli both have anti-prostate tumor properties but the combination is better than the sum of the effects individually[246]. Eating two different fruits together has a greater antioxidant capacity than the same amount of either fruit consumed individually[247]. Vitamin C helps to make iron more absorbable so a combination of fruit with iron-containing vegetables (leeks, beet greens, kale, spinach, etc.) may be particularly effective for this purpose[248].

PSYCHOLOGICAL STRESS AND INFLAMMATION

Major stressful life events are large risk factors for the emergence of a clinical depression[249]. For example, life events involving social rejection alone could result in a 22% increase in

---

[246] The reason for this enhancement is unknown; Canene-Adams, K., Lindshield, B., Wang, S., Jeffery, E., Clinton, S., & Erdman, J. (2007). Combinations of Tomato and Broccoli Enhance Antitumor Activity in Dunning R3327-H Prostate Adenocarcinomas. *Cancer Research, 67,* 836-843.

[247] Liu, R. (2003). Health benefits of fruit and vegetables are from additive and synergistic combinations of phytochemicals. The American Journal of Clinical Nutrition, 78(3), 517S-520S.

[248] Weber, J., & Zimmerman, M. (2009). The men's health big book of food & nutrition: Your completely delicious guide to eating well, looking great, and staying lean for life! (p. 102). New York: Rodale.

[249] Kendler, K. S., Karkowski, L. M., & Prescott, C. A. (1999). Causal relationship between stressful life events and the onset of major depression. *American Journal of Psychiatry, 156,* 837-848.

risk for onset of a depressive disorder[250]. Exposure to recent major life stress (cognitive upheaval and disruption to a person's goals, plans, and aspirations) is considered to be a strong risk factor for depression, with up to 80% of depressive episodes in the general population being precipitated by such stress[251].

There is now substantial evidence that psychological stress can trigger significant increases in inflammatory activity[252]. So our physical environmental/ social conditions and perhaps even more importantly our *perception and interpretation* of those conditions may have a direct neurobiological effect that increases the risk for depression. Moreover, these processes may also influence the development of other disease conditions that have an inflammatory basis and tend to co-occur with depression, such as vascular disease, chronic pain, obesity, and diabetes.

Two physiological pathways are responsible for converting environmental/ social – or their negative interpretation – into inflammatory responses. The first pathway involves the *sympathetic nervous system* and the second the so-called *hypothalamic-pituitary-adrenal* (HPA) axis.

---

[250] Kendler, K. S., Hettema, J. M., Butera, F.. Gardner, C. O., & Prescott, C. A. (2003). Life event dimensions of loss, humiliation, entrapment, and danger in the prediction of onsets of major depression and generalized anxiety. *Archives of General Psychiatry, 60,* 789-796. doi: lO.lOOl/archpsyc.60.8.789.

[251] Mazure, C. M. (1998). Life Stressors as risk factors in depression. *Clinical Psychology: Science and Practice, 5,* 291-313. doi:10.1111/j.1468-2850 .1998.tbOO151.x.

[252] Glaser, R., & Kiecolt-Glaser, J. K. (2005). Stress-induced immune dysfunction: Implications for health. Nature Reviews Immunology, 5, 243- 251. doi: 10.1038/nri 1571.

From an evolutionary standpoint, environmental stress was primarily an acute attack by predators or pathogens that led to activation of the innate immune response involving the sympathetic nervous system and cytokine production that enhances wound healing and physical recovery. Acute activation of the HPA axis triggers cortisol (adrenaline) secretion that allows instant focus of all energy and attention to the invader. Normally there is a balance between cortisol and cytokines, the cortisol being anti-inflammatory and the cytokines inflammatory. However, contemporary "threats" are usually psychosocial perceptions that tend to be more prolonged than actual physical threats for which the system was designed. Under these conditions, cortisol receptors become less sensitive and allow an unbalanced inflammatory response.

Such inflammation can then lead to oxidative stress, and vice versa. Therefore, psychological stress can lead to both inflammation and physiologic oxidative stress.

While we shall focus on diet – what you put into your mouth, what you put into your head, that is to say your thinking, is also important, as is exercise, sleep, and a number of other factors.

Techniques for controlling your thinking are of critical importance to reduce psychological stress. A best practice for doing that is *cognitive behavioral therapy* (CBT). Although the focus of this book is reducing psychological stress and treatment of the neurobiological consequences of stress through diet, we include in Chapter 19 the basics of CBT. In addition to lowering psychological stress, the same techniques are useful in changing habits and addictions such as those pertaining to one's diet.

PLANT STRESS RESPONSE CAN ASSIST HUMAN STRESS RESPONSE: XENOHORMESIS

The phenomenon whereby a "foreign" organism's stress response yields benefits to another organism is called xenohormesis[253]. This refers most often to stressed plants producing compounds conferring stress tolerance to animals that consume them. This is even more remarkable when one considers that the mechanism of reaction to stress is completely different in plants versus animals.

Plants manufacture thousands of substances in response to stress from heat and cold, fungal, viral, bacterial, and insect attacks, water deficiencies, and many other stressors. The table below lists a few such examples of xenohormesis.

Figure 5 Xenohormesis

Plant	Stressor	Bioactive Product	Benefit to human
Cucumber	fungal and viral infection	salicylate	vascular disease
Tumeric	nutrient deprevation, heat stress	curcumin	mood disorders
Dandelion	inhibition of DNA repair	phenolic compounds	antioxidants, anti-inflammatory
Grape	heat	phenolic compounds	antioxidants, anti-inflammatory
Green Algae	light and nutrient stress	carotenoids	vascular disease
Lettuce	Heat, cold, light stress	ascorbic acid, phenolic compounds	antioxidants, anti-inflammatory
Oregano	bacterial infection	varvacrol	anti-inflammatory
St. John's wort	water deficit	hyperforin	anti-depressant
Strawberry	water deficit	phenolic compounds	antioxidants, anti-inflammatory
Willow seedlings	beetles	salicylate	vascular disease

---

[253] Howitz KT, Sinclair DA (2008) Xenohormesis: sensing the chemical cues of other species. Cell 133:387–391.

Cucumber and willow seedlings use salicylate to fight fungi/ viral infections and beetle invasion, while humans use the same substance as an anti-inflammatory; although this anti- inflammatory has been used as a manufactured substance (aspirin, see Chapter 5, with its side effects including possible death), most plants have this and many other anti- inflammatories. Thus whole plants are a better choice than manufactured isolated anti-inflammatories, or at least a safe supplemental choice.

Turmeric produces curcumin, in plants for nutrient deprivation and heat stress; in humans, it serves as a powerful antioxidant and anti-inflammatory, among other healthful benefits.

Dandelions, a bitter plant considered by most a weed to be avoided, produces phenolic compounds that are protective to DNA damage in the plant and are very strong anti-oxidants and anti-inflammatories in humans.

Phenolic compounds are also produced in grapes and strawberries in response to heat and water-deficit stressors.

Green algae produce carotenoids to alleviate stress from light and lower nutrient sources and are useful in humans for vascu- lar disease and other stressors.

When St. John's wort is stressed by lack of water, it increases the bioactive compound hyperforin, the active molecular spe- cies assisting clinical depression.

The point here is that plants are super anti-oxidant producers by necessity and we can utilize this by their consumption. As we shall see, plants and plant parts that have the most surface area in direct contact with the sun tend to have the most anti- oxidants; this is true of most green leafy plants, particularly the darker ones that absorb the most energy in the visible spectrum from the sun. The leaves are like edible solar energy cells that track the sun.

RELATIONSHIP OF OXIDATIVE STRESS AND INFLAMMATION

During the activation of the innate inflammatory process, specialized cellular components in the blood, called *mast cells* and *leukocytes*, are recruited to the site of damage, leading to a "respiratory burst" due to an increased uptake of oxygen, and thus, an increased release and accumulation of free radicals at the site of damage[254][255].

The immune system uses the lethal effects of oxidants by utilizing the production of oxidizing species as a central part of its mechanism of killing pathogens; with foreign invading material being ingested by cells called *phagocytes* that produce both reactive oxidizing and reactive nitrogen species[256][257].

---

[254] Hussain, S. P., Hofseth, L. J., & Harris, C. C. (2003). Radical causes of cancer.*Nature Reviews Cancer Nat Rev Cancer, 3*(4), 276-285. doi:10.1038/nrc1046.

[255] Coussens, L. M., & Werb, Z. (2002). Inflammation and cancer. *Nature, 420*(6917), 860-867. doi:10.1038/nature01322.

[256] Nathan, C., & Shiloh, M. U. (2000). Reactive oxygen and nitrogen intermediates in the relationship between mammalian hosts and microbial pathogens. *Proceedings of the National Academy of Sciences, 97*(16), 8841-8848. doi:10.1073/pnas.97.16.8841.

[257] Maes, M., Mihaylova, I., Kubera, M., Uytterhoeven, M., Vrydags, N., & Bosmans, E. (2010). Increased plasma peroxides and serum oxidized low density lipoprotein antibodies in major depression: Markers that further explain the higher incidence of neurodegeneration and coronary artery disease. *Journal of Affective Disorders, 125*(1-3), 287-294. doi:10.1016/j.jad.2009.12.014.

On the other hand, recent research has revealed the mechanism by which continued oxidative stress can lead to chronic inflammation. For example, oxidative stress is thought to be linked to vascular disease since oxidation of LDL in the vascular endothelium is a precursor to plaque formation.

OXIDATIVE STRESS AND MENTAL DISORDERS

Numerous physiological and pathological processes such as aging, excessive caloric intake, infections, inflammatory disorders, environmental toxins, pharmacological treatments, emotional or psychological stress, ionizing radiation, cigarette smoke and excessive alcohol consumption increase the bodily concentration of oxidizing substances.

There are many biomarkers employed as indices of oxidative stress correlated with the existence of mental disorders. These have been found, for example, in child and adolescent patients diagnosed with attention deficit/ hyperactivity disorder[258], in adults with bipolar disorder[259], and in patients with paranoid schizophrenia[260] as well as mood disorders such as clinical depression. Oxidative stress has been found also to

> *Psychological stress is inflammatory.*

---

[258] Ceylan, M. F., Sener, S., Bayraktar, A. C., & Kavutcu, M. (2012). Changes in oxidative stress and cellular immunity serum markers in attention-deficit/hyperactivity disorder. Psychiatry and Clinical Neurosciences, 66, 220–226. doi:10.1111/j.1440-1819.2012.02330.x.

[259] Andreazza, A. C., Kauer-Sant'anna, M., Frey, B. N., Bond, D. J., Kapczinski, F., Young, L. T., & Yatham, L. N. (2008). Oxidative stress markers in bipolar disorder: A metaanalysis. Journal of Affective Disorders, 111, 135–144. doi:10.1016/j.jad.2008.04.013.

[260] Dietrich-Muszalska, A., Malinowska, J., Olas, B., Glowacki, R., Bald, E., Wachowicz, B., & Rabe-Jablonska, J. (2012). The oxidative stress may be induced by the elevated homocysteine in schizophrenic patients. Neurochemical Research, 37, 1057–1062. doi:10.1007/s11064-012-0707-3.

be indirectly associated with anxiety disorders; mental retardation, autistic spectrum disorder, Rett's disorder, delirium, dementia related disorders, eating disorders, and sleep disorders[261].

Stress is associated with a range of psychiatric problems.

Oxidative stress has been found to be higher in individuals with depression, whereas antioxidant capacity is lower[262]. Intakes of beta carotene, vitamin C, fiber, and folate—nutrients found in fruits and vegetables—have been shown to be lower in those with depression compared to individuals without depression[263]. Note that while whole-plant food-derived phytochemicals have been associated with mental health benefits, antioxidants from dietary supplements extracted from plants appear to be less beneficial and may, in fact, be detrimental to health[264].

One cross-sectional study with control group summarized[265]:

---

[261] Tsaluchidu, S., Cocchi, M., Tonello, L., & Puri, B. K. (2008). Fatty acids and oxidative stress in psychiatric disorders. *BMC Psychiatry, 8*(Suppl 1). doi:10.1186/1471-244x-8-s1-s5.

[262] Kodydková, J., Vávrová, L., Zeman, M., Jirák, R., Macášek, J., Staňková, B., . . . Žák, A. (2009). Antioxidative enzymes and increased oxidative stress in depressive women. *Clinical Biochemistry, 42*(13-14), 1368-1374. doi:10.1016/j.clinbiochem.2009.06.006.

[263] Park, J., You, J., & Chang, K. (2010). Dietary taurine intake, nutrients intake, dietary habits and life stress by depression in Korean female college students: A case-control study. *J Biomed Sci Journal of Biomedical Science, 17*(Suppl 1). doi:10.1186/1423-0127-17-s1-s40.

[264] Bjelakovic, G., Nikolova, D., Gluud, L. L., Simonetti, R. G., & Gluud, C. (2007). Mortality in Randomized Trials of Antioxidant Supplements for Primary and Secondary Prevention. *Jama, 297*(8), 842. doi:10.1001/jama.297.8.842.

[265] Payne, M. E., Steck, S. E., George, R. R., & Steffens, D. C. (2012). Fruit, Vegetable, and Antioxidant Intakes Are Lower in Older Adults with

"Intakes of fruits, vegetables, and naturally occurring antioxidants, specifically vitamin C and beta cryptoxanthin, were found to be inversely associated with depression in this sample of elderly patients with depression and comparison participants, although no association was found with antioxidant supplements."

Therefore, many studies suggest likely merit in a change of diet to one that is rich in free radical scavengers. There is already strong epidemiological rodent and human evidence that a change in diet to a primarily a whole-food varied-plant diet devoid of refined carbohydrate products may help prevent and possibly even reverse certain mental disorders.

NEURONAL REGENERATION IN THE ADULT

Contrary to old beliefs, brain tissue can regenerate in certain areas of the brain, the main area being in the hippocampus. That area of the brain is particularly sensitive to the biochemistry of stress, and chronic stress reduces neuroregeneration and can reduce hippocampal size. These effects show up in severe clinical depression[266], post-traumatic stress disorder[267], and schizophrenia[268].

Depression. *Journal of the Academy of Nutrition and Dietetics, 112*(12), 2022-2027. doi:10.1016/j.jand.2012.08.026.

[266] Kempton, M. J. (2011). Structural Neuroimaging Studies in Major Depressive Disorder. *Arch Gen Psychiatry Archives of General Psychiatry, 68*(7), 675. doi:10.1001/archgenpsychiatry.2011.60.

[267] Karl A, Schaefer M, Malta LS, Dörfel D, Rohleder N, Werner A (2006). "A meta-analysis of structural brain abnormalities in PTSD". *Neuroscience and Biobehavioral Reviews.* **30** (7): 1004–31.

Antidepressants appear to help reverse this process by inducing neurogenesis with consequent improvement of symptoms of depression and anxiety. This could explain the two to six week delayed onset of antidepressant action, the time taken for significant neurogenesis to occur[269].

But also dietary polyphenols seem to exert positive effects on anxiety and depression, in part by increase in adult hippocampal neurogenesis. Studies on the effects of dietary polyphenols on behavior may play an important role in the approach to use diet as part of the therapeutic interventions for mental health.

Dietary polyphenols are most abundant in antioxidants[270]. This has been shown in a diet based on the combination of polyphenols from blueberries and green tea, as well as antioxidant and anti-inflammatory amino acids like carnosine[271].

One animal study revealed that polyphenols from flaxseeds with omega-3 fatty acids were able to reduce all chronic mild stress symptoms.

---

[268] Wright, I. C., Rabe-Hesketh, S., Woodruff, P. W., David, A. S., Murray, R. M., & Bullmore, E. T. (2000). Meta-Analysis of Regional Brain Volumes in Schizophrenia. *American Journal of Psychiatry AJP, 157*(1), 16-25. doi:10.1176/ajp.157.1.16.

[269] Malberg JE, Eisch AJ, Nestler EJ, Duman RS. (2000). Chronic antidepressant treatment increases neurogenesis in adult rat hippocampus. J Neurosci 20:9104 – 9110.

[270] Scalbert A & Williamson G (2000) Dietary intake and bioavailability of polyphenols. J Nutr 130, 2073S–2085S.

[271] Acosta, S., Jernberg, J., Sanberg, C., Sanberg, P., Small, B. J., Gemma, C., & Bickford, P. C. (2010). NT-020, a Natural Therapeutic Approach to Optimize Spatial Memory Performance and Increase Neural Progenitor Cell Proliferation and Decrease Inflammation in the Aged Rat. *Rejuvenation Research, 13*(5), 581-588. doi:10.1089/rej.2009.1011.

Note the mechanisms for positive polyphenol effects on mental health are not limited to their well-established antioxidant effects and are as varied as the different polyphenols themselves and the sources in which they are found. For example, *chlorogenic acid* is a common dietary polyphenol found in fruits such as plums, apples, and cherries and beverages such as tea and coffee, which has been shown to have anti-depressive and anxiolytic properties[272].

MITOCHONDRIAL DISORDER AND MENTAL DISORDER

As we have previously explored, the mitochondrion is the power source for each cell in our body. Gene mutations in mitochondrial DNA that impair mitochondrial function and result in deficient energy production can give rise to clinical syndromes[273]. Mitochondrial disorders typically present with multiple symptoms affecting highly energy-dependent tissues such as muscle and the brain. Psychiatric illness may be the presenting feature of a mitochondrial disorder.

The most common psychiatric presentations in the cases of mitochondrial disorders included mood disorder, cognitive deterioration, psychosis, and anxiety[274].

---

[272] Manach C., Scalbert A., Morand C., Rémésy C., Jimenez L. (2004). Polyphenols: food sources and bioavailability. Am. J. Clin. Nutr. 79, 727–747.

[273] Dimauro, S., & Schon, E. A. (2003). Mitochondrial Respiratory-Chain Diseases.*New England Journal of Medicine N Engl J Med, 348*(26).

[274] Anglin, R. E., et al.(2012). The Psychiatric Manifestations of Mitochondrial Disorders. *J. Clin. Psychiatry The Journal of Clinical Psychiatry, 73*(04), 506-512. doi:10.4088/jcp.11r07237.

CHAPTER 7

Gut Feelings

"Trust your gut. "

THE GUT-BRAIN AXIS

We are understanding that genetics is not our destiny. Perhaps the two newest and most exciting illustrations of this fact are epigenetics, where genes are switched "on and off" by extra-genomic variation, and our intestinal microbiome, a community of social microorganisms in our gut influenced by our diet and communicating with our brain.[275].

Consider the amazing fact that most of the cells in our bodies are not human: they are microbial cells, mainly bacteria that

---

[275] Tuohy, K., Gougoulias, C., Shen, Q., Walton, G., Fava, F., & Ramnani, P. (2009). Studying the Human Gut Microbiota in the Trans-Omics Era - Focus on Metagenomics and Metabonomics. CPD Current Pharmaceutical Design, 15(13), 1415-1427. doi:10.2174/138161209788168182.

constitute our microbiome. The "typical" human is comprised of about 30 trillion human cells and 39 trillion bacteria[276] with 40,000 microbial species[277]. There is a symbiotic relationship we have with microorganisms, as do all animals and all plants (refer back to an aforementioned early symbiosis of eukaryotic cells forming the mitochondria and later chloroplasts for cellular energy).

The so-called *gut-brain axis* is the biochemical signaling system between the gastrointestinal (GI) tract and the central nervous system (CNS). This microbiome is an integral part of this communication. In addition to the central nervous system and the GI tract, the gut - brain axis includes neuroendocrine and neuroimmune systems and the *enteric nervous system* (ENS). The ENS communicates with the CNS but can act independently; it has been referred to as a "second brain[278]."

There is a bi-directional influence of our microbiome and our brain.

The importance of emotional states and stress processing in the brain has been recognized for some time in the etiology of gastric ulcer formation and generally with the exacerbation of GI disturbances, but the bidirectional nature of the gut-brain axis is becoming more appreciated recently. There is little doubt that emotional distress is associated with GI dysfunction

---

276 Sender, R., Fuchs, S., & Milo, R. (2016). Revised estimates for the number of human and bacteria cells in the body. doi:10.1101/036103.

277 Frank, D. N., & Pace, N. R. (2008). Gastrointestinal microbiology enters the metagenomics era. *Current Opinion in Gastroenterology, 24*(1), 4-10. doi:10.1097/mog.0b013e3282f2b0e8.

278 Li, Y., & Owyang, C. (2003). Musings on the Wanderer: What's New in Our Understanding of Vago-Vagal Reflexes? V. Remodeling of vagus and enteric neural circuitry after vagal injury. *American Journal of Physiology - Gastrointestinal and Liver Physiology Am J Physiol Gastrointest Liver Physiol,285*(3). doi:10.1152/ajpgi.00119.2003.

and vice versa. But the association is much more connected than previously thought.

Most bacterial cells reside in the GI system, primarily the colon, where they protect the intestinal barrier defense system, digest our food, extract the nutrients that we need, and in some cases synthesize nutrients[279] for their human host. This ecological community in the GI tract is an integral part of the system of bidirectional communication between the gut and the brain.

An imbalance in gut bacteria (*dysbiosis*) and disruption of the integrity of the gut barrier, can lead to the induction of inflammatory responses[280] including mood disorders. One possible cause of gut dysbiosis is depletion from the environment of microorganisms with which humans co-evolved.

The so-called *hygiene hypothesis*, or "old friends theory" states that a reduced exposure from birth to the microorganisms accompanying mammalian evolution, for example associated with the vaginal birth canal, feces, animals and mud, suppresses the natural development of the immune system. It is thought that this reduced microbial exposure leads to chronic inflammatory diseases such as depression[281]. This does correlate on a time scale consistent with the increasing

---

[279] Carpenter, S. (2012). That gut feeling: Exploring the mind-belly-bacteria connection. *Monitor on Psychology, 43*, 51–55.

[280] Berk, M., Williams, L. J., Jacka, F. N., O'Neil, A., Pasco, J. A., Moylan, S., . . . Byrne, M. L. (2013). So depression is an inflammatory disease, but where does the inflammation come from? *BMC Medicine, 11*, 200. Retrieved from http:// www.biomedcentral.com/1741-7015/11/200.

[281] Raison, C. L., Lowry, C. A., & Rook, G. A. (2010). Inflammation, Sanitation, and Consternation. *Arch Gen Psychiatry Archives of General Psychiatry, 67*(12), 1211. doi:10.1001/archgenpsychiatry.2010.161.

incidence of mood disorders in the "post-hygienic" era of Western societies since the late nineteenth century.

PSYCHIATRIC DISORDERS AND THE GUT-BRAIN AXIS

Mystical interpretations of mental illness over the centuries were largely replaced in the nineteenth century with institutionalization into asylums; the classic Greek theory of "humors" or bodily fluids causing mental disturbances if in an "imbalance" was re-adopted. Most popular amongst the humor adjustments was the 2000 year old practice of bloodletting, modelled after the process of menstruation thought to "purge woman of bad humors[282]."

However, psychiatry as an early field of medicine struggled as the symptoms, often dramatic, typically had an unclear etiology. There arose a division in thinking of psychiatric illness in the late nineteenth century as being "organic" and "functional." Organic mental illness had some possible physical basis such as following a head injury or infection. Functional illness was thought to arise in the mind, distinct from the neurochemical workings of the brain. This was supported by the emergence of psychoanalytic approach of Dr. Freud with his "talking cure."

For a brief period of time in the early twentieth century there was exploration of the possible medical basis for psychiatric disorders otherwise considered "functional" illnesses.

For example, consider the work of Henry A. Cotton, MD. In his 1921 text *The Defective Delinquent and the Insane*[283], he

---

[282] Coutinho, E. M., Segal, S. J., & Coutinho, E. M. (1999). *Is menstruation obsolete?* New York: Oxford University Press.

[283] Cotton, Henry A., M .D. Medical Director New Jersey State Hospital, Trenton, U.S.A. The Defective Delinquent and Insane. Oxford University Press, 1921.

explored topics such as "biological considerations of the nature of insanity, indirect actions of physical disorders on the brain," and causes of mental illness from "disturbances of the endocrine system," and "chronic infections." He wrote[284]:

> *"While psychiatrists, in the past, have held the non-biological view of the nature of the so-called functional mental disturbances, the biologists have produced evidence regarding function and structure which when applied to mental disorders will, undoubtedly, modify these traditional ideas. The biologists are definite in the assertion that there can be no function without structure. This being true it would also be true that there can be no abnormal function without a corresponding abnormal structure. Medical men have been willing to admit this fundamental law so far as it related to other organs in the body but there has been some hesitancy in accepting this truth when applied to the brain and the mind."*

His primary interest on healing mental disorders was on disturbances in the immune system through chronic infections and toxins local to the teeth and the GI system. Treatment involved the use of antibiotics (recently being revisited as a treatment for mood disorders[285]) and resection of portions of the large and small intestines. This was an early type of "psychosurgery."

---

[284] Ibid, p 14.
[285] Antibiotics for Affective Disorders - Focus on Minocycline. (2016). *Bipolar Disorders, 18*16-17. doi:10.1111/bdi.12404.

Psychosurgery was popular just prior to the first effective pharmacologic interventions. The first type of psychosurgery was colectomy – removal of part of the small intestine or colon. The theory was that[286]

> *"If the infection is limited to certain areas, segmental in character, it may be possible to remove such infection by resection. Marked improvement in the mental symptoms has repeatedly been observed following such a procedure. If, however, the infection is very extensive, involving more of the bowel than is considered wise to remove, the disease must be attacked either by vaccine or serum. This is especially true when evidence of infection is found to extend throughout the whole length of the small intestine. In these cases, the administration of specific antistreptococcic and anti-colon bacillus serum, made from strains isolated in the laboratory of the State Hospital, has proven very successful."*

As indicated earlier in Chapter 2, effective treatments for psychiatric illness didn't blossom until the middle of the twentieth century with the development of plant-derived alkaloids; first Thorazine for psychosis and then its derivative, imipramine, for depression.

---

[286] Cotton, p.18.

ATTENTION DEFICIT HYPERACTIVITY DISORDERS *(ADHD)*

The gut microbiota is known to participate in susceptibility to allergies, especially food allergens[287]. One meta-analysis reported that the elimination of salicylates, artificial food colors and flavors, and preservatives could decrease the hyperactivity of children with ADHD[288]. Children with ADHD also substantially improved with dietary supplementations of polyunsaturated fatty acids, iron, and zinc[289]. Food-based treatments in children with allergic disorders have been shown to significantly reduce ADHD-like behavior[290].

THE INTESTINAL EPITHELIUM

The most precarious barrier between the outside world and our inside body is a single layer of cells lining the gut called the intestinal epithelium. These cells are "selectively" permeable, i.e., they let into the body nutrients from our diet but block the passage of microorganisms and toxins. Should that system fail, an immune response is stimulated and this is communicated to

---

[287] Cao, S., Feehley, T. J., & Nagler, C. R. (2014). The role of commensal bacteria in the regulation of sensitization to food allergens. *FEBS Letters, 588*(22), 4258-4266. doi:10.1016/j.febslet.2014.04.026.

[288] Schab, D. W., & Trinh, N. T. (2004). Do Artificial Food Colors Promote Hyperactivity in Children with Hyperactive Syndromes? A Meta-Analysis of Double-Blind Placebo-Controlled Trials. *Journal of Developmental & Behavioral Pediatrics, 25*(6), 423-434. doi:10.1097/00004703-200412000-00007.

[289] Murphy, E. F., Cotter, P. D., Healy, S., Marques, T. M., O'sullivan, O., Fouhy, F., . . . Shanahan, F. (2010). Composition and energy harvesting capacity of the gut microbiota: Relationship to diet, obesity and time in mouse models. *Gut, 59*(12), 1635-1642. doi:10.1136/gut.2010.215665.

[290] Theije, C. G., Bavelaar, B. M., Silva, S. L., Korte, S. M., Olivier, B., Garssen, J., & Kraneveld, A. D. (2013). Food allergy and food-based therapies in neurodevelopmental disorders. *Pediatric Allergy and Immunology, 25*(3), 218-226. doi:10.1111/pai.12149.

the brain, influencing mood[291]. Intestinal permeability is influenced by a number of factors including diet, alcohol, medications such as non-steroidal anti-inflammatories, and physical or psychological stress.

> *Inflammation of the gut, as results from animal endotoxins, can have psychiatric implications.*

LEAKY GUT

A single meal high in animal fat causes an immediate elevation in inflammation that can be measured, for example, by a restriction in blood flow in arteries through our body[292] maximizing in about 4 hours and recovering in five or six hours. The reason for this is the existence of bacterial endotoxins after a meal of meat, eggs, or dairy[293].

PSYCHOBIOTICS

We shall define psychobiotics as live micro-organisms which, when administered in adequate amounts, confer a cognitive or emotional health benefit on the host through changes in the gut microbiota.

---

[291] Groschwitz, K. R., & Hogan, S. P. (2009). Intestinal barrier function: Molecular regulation and disease pathogenesis. *Journal of Allergy and Clinical Immunology, 124*(1), 3-20. doi:10.1016/j.jaci.2009.05.038.

[292] Vogel, R. A., Corretti, M. C., & Plotnick, G. D. (1997). Effect of a Single High-Fat Meal on Endothelial Function in Healthy Subjects. *The American Journal of Cardiology, 79*(3), 350-354. doi:10.1016/s0002-9149(96)00760-6.

[293] Deopurkar, R., Ghanim, H., Friedman, J., Abuaysheh, S., Sia, C. L., Mohanty, P., . . . Dandona, P. (2010). Differential Effects of Cream, Glucose, and Orange Juice on Inflammation, Endotoxin, and the Expression of Toll-Like Receptor-4 and Suppressor of Cytokine Signaling-3. *Diabetes Care, 33*(5), 991-997. doi:10.2337/dc09-1630.

Thomas Insel, Director of the National Institute of Mental Health, referred to recent studies on the microbiota as among the most important recently published in the field of psychiatry and concluded that[294]

> *"Our bodies are ... a complex ecosystem in which human cells represent a paltry 10% of the population. But beyond the sheer numbers, we now know about the profound diversity of this ecosystem and striking individual differences. How these differences in our microbial world influence the development of brain and behavior will be one of the great frontiers of clinical neuroscience in the next decade."*

There is an expanding volume of evidence to support the view that cognitive and emotional processes can be altered by microbes acting through the brain-gut axis in a bi-directional manner. An exciting active area of research is to analyze ones microbiome and adjust it for cognitive and emotional wellness.

The first published proposal for the use of probiotics as adjunct therapy in the management of depression was detailed in 2005[295]. Psychobiotics may function mechanistically as delivery vehicles for neuroactive compounds acting as psychotropic agents[296]. It is clear that a broad range of bacteria manufacture

---

[294] Insel T (2012): National Institute of Mental Health. Director's Blog. Available at: http://www.nimh.nih.gov/about/director/index.shtml. Accessed January 15, 2013.

[295] Logan, A. C., & Katzman, M. (2005). Major depressive disorder: Probiotics may be an adjuvant therapy. *Medical Hypotheses, 64*(3), 533-538. doi:10.1016/j.mehy.2004.08.019.

[296] Lyte, M. (2011). Probiotics function mechanistically as delivery vehicles for neuroactive compounds: Microbial endocrinology in the design

and secrete neurochemicals and this is another possible mechanism of influence on the central nervous system. For example, certain strains of Lactobacillus and Bifidobacterium secrete gamma-aminobutyric acid (GABA), which has a direct influence on anxiety and depression[297].

Clinical studies thus far are few. In one double-blind, placebo-controlled, randomized parallel group study, volunteers received either a psychobiotic combination or placebo. Daily administration of the psychobiotic combination significantly reduced psychological distress, anxiety and depression[298].

The future may bring dietary psychobiotics that optimize gut flora for emotional health.

Another study[299] found that the consumption of a psychobiotic improved mood in one hundred twenty-four participants. Clinical research on a group of patients with chronic fatigue syndrome were treated three times daily with Lactobacillus casei strain Shirota or a placebo with identical taste and appearance[300]. Overall, there was a

---

and use of probiotics. *BioEssays, 33*(8), 574-581. doi:10.1002/bies.201100024.

[297] Schousboe A, Waagepetersen HS (2007): GABA: Homeostatic and pharmacological aspects. In: Tepper JM, Abercrombie ED, Bolam JP, editors. GABA and the Basal Ganglia: From Molecules to Systems. Amsterdam: Elsevier Science Bv, 9–19.

[298] Messaoudi M, Lalonde R, Violle N, Javelot H, Desor D, Nejdi A, et al. (2011): Assessment of psychotropic-like properties of a probiotic formulation (Lactobacillus helveticus R0052 and Bifidobacterium longum R0175) in rats and human subjects. Br J Nutr 105:755–764.

[299] Benton D, Williams C, Brown A (2007): Impact of consuming a milk drink containing a probiotic on mood and cognition. Eur J Clin Nutr 61: 355–361.

[300] Rao AV, Bested AC, Beaulne TM, Katzman MA, Iorio C, Berardi JM, Logan AC (2009): A randomized, double-blind, placebo-controlled pilot

significant improvement in anxiety among those taking the active psychobiotics compared to the placebo, providing further support for the view that a probiotic may have psychotropic effects.

The gut microbiota is a complex metabolic ecosystem and when adults ingest probiotics, such bacteria usually transit the gut or transiently colonize rather than becoming a permanent feature[301]. Therefore, it is likely that if effective psychobiotics are identified, they would need to be adopted into a dietary pattern rather than creating a permanently altered microbiome.

However, in this newly developing field of the brain-gut connection, no current recommendation for dietary interventions can be made for psychobiotics to improve cognition and emotion. Expectations are high for the near future.

---

study of a probiotic in emotional symptoms of chronic fatigue syndrome. Gut Pathog 1:6.

[301] Alander M, Satokari R, Korpela R, Saxelin M, Vilpponen-Salmela T, Mattila-Sandholm vonWright A (1999): Persistence of colonization of human colonic mucosa by a probiotic strain, Lactobacillus rhamnosus GG, after oral consumption. Appl Environ Microbiol 65:351–354.

Part III WHAT

What food is best for health and happiness? In the section we shall detail what to eat and the science behind the suggestions.

CHAPTER 8

The Science and Art of Nutrition

"One should eat to live, not live to eat."

Molière

FOOD AS ART

Art is difficult to define but simply put, it is the appreciated product of creative human play. Play in the sense of Mark Twain:

> *"Work consists of whatever a body is obliged to do. Play consists of whatever a body is not obliged to do."*

Using this definition, art is a relatively new hominid concept, at least at the level of current appreciation. Art relates first to the senses, then the emotions - often by association. The sense of sound lends itself to music, vision to the visual arts, and touch to tactile physical stimulation. A sentiment of some individuals in advanced societies is: *the earth without art is "eh"*[302].

What about taste? Taste remains as the most primitive of senses with its basic function of survival. Eating has been our most important activity, besides procreating, and food source selection has been based for the most part on taste.

Today, we have identified safe food sources, highly reducing the critical function of taste for survival. The evolutionary adaptation of taste may be divided into two types: bitter and sweet. These taste fibers are hardwired at the brainstem level. There have now been identified additional taste receptors for different nuances of taste that do not appear fundamental to our genetic make-up, such as salty, sour, and savory or umami.

These relatively recent taste sensations have a role in the artistic development of culinary art, but likely a minor one, compared to the advancement of smell. Primates have never had the sensitive sense of smell that many other animals have of their external environment, but there is another advanced type of smell involved in human appreciation of food that surpasses all other animals: this smell is involved with the appreciation of flavor.

---

[302] If this is not obvious, subtract the letters "art" from the word earth leaving the remaining letters "eh" a colloquialism for blandness.

NEUROGASTRONOMY[303]

There are two very different neurochemical pathways involved in human perception of smell: exterior or frontal smell, also called *orthonasal* smell, similar in many other animals, and posterior or *retronasal* smell. This latter type of smell is much different from the former: it has receptor fibers for volatile gases that directly connect to the frontal cortex, a highly intellectual area of the brain. It is this retronasal smell, combined with taste, that leads to the artistic realm of flavor.

If one judges a food to "taste good", that person is making judgment on its flavor. This is an important finding. Tastes are rather fixed; most everyone has similar perception of sweet and bitter, for example, although there are varying sensitivities among individuals. However *flavor*, being an interpretive higher cognitive function, can be influenced by association[304].

> *Taste has been important in our survival as a species. However, now flavor has replaced taste as our motivation for food selection.*

Much of the brain is integrated. Neuronal fibers from the smell regions of the frontal cortex communicate with diverse areas of the brain having to do with memory, emotion, and behavior. There are also connections to various other areas of the prefrontal cortex involved in learning and decisions about rewards, so-called *executive function*. Even the way food looks (presentation) and feels in our mouth

---

[303] Much of this section is based on facts presented by Shepherd, G. (2013). *Neurogastronomy: How the brain creates flavor and why it matters* (Reprint ed.). New York: Columbia University Press.

[304] We shall use the word *taste* as a noun to mean the sensations of the sweet, sour, bitter, or salty quality of a food. Taste or tasting as a verb will be taken to mean to sense the flavor of a food.

(texture) have some influence on the overall perception of flavor.

These advanced brain regions are not fully developed until well into adulthood, perhaps explaining the culinary reluctance and more limited dietary patterns of children and adolescents.

That flavor is highly influenced by retronasal smell is evident to anyone with a "stuffy nose". This can also be simulated by pinching the nose or by mouth breathing only. This does not affect the taste receptors so can be an interesting experiment to detect, for example, bitter and sweet taste thresholds without the influence of flavor.

FOOD AS SURVIVAL

Flavor can be a beautiful thing and is the basis for the culinary arts. But it shouldn't *always* be the basis of one's diet – that should still be survival, and that means selection of nutrient-dense foods in addition to some energy-dense foods.

Consider the analogous situation for the other senses. For example, we enjoy hearing beautiful music but usually use our sense of hearing for more practical purposes. Similarly, we may enjoy the visual arts but primarily use the sense of vision in a utilitarian way, as for safety.

To rethink one's flavor and overall taste associations, we offer a cognitive behavioral approach in Chapter 19.

All nutrients – macronutrients and micronutrients - come from plants reacting with the sun. If we eat animals or animal products, that food may or may not have some of the nutrients we need but they contain compounds we don't need – and shouldn't want.

We have detailed in another book, titled *The New Ancestral Diet*[305], from an analysis of the past 85 million years of primate history, how we have evolved on a diet of whole-food varied-plants. Only very recently in our history as a species have we begun to eat energy-dense animals, first by scavenging organs and marrow and then, after control of fire, cooking and consuming flesh.

Genetic metabolic changes occurred in our direct ancestors tens of millions of years ago including losing our ability to self-manufacture the following essential micronutrients:

- thiamine
- riboflavin
- niacin
- vitamin A
- vitamin C

Over the millennia we also lost the ability to produce substances such as alpha gal (two million years ago) and Neu5Gc (20 million years ago)[306]. Those were useful adaptations at the time; unfortunately, mammals other than those directly in our lineage still make these substances but our bodies treat them as pathologic substances. The alpha gal allergy is also known as "meat-allergy[307]." These compounds are involved in immune activation leading to chronic inflammation and autoimmune disorders, including cancers.

---

[305] Aiken R.C. & Aiken, D.C. (2015) *The new ancestral diet*. Go-Ahead Publishing, Los Angeles.

[306] The alpha gal story is an interesting one; search this phrase on Dr. Michael Greger's informative website NutritionFacts.org.

[307] Fulmer, M. L. (2013). Galactose-alpha-1,3-galactose: Possible Role in Red Meat Allergy. *J Biosafety Health Educ Journal of Biosafety & Health Education, 01*(04). doi:10.4172/2332-0893.1000e110.

As discussed in Chapter 5, we know that meat contains bacteria that produce endotoxins taken up by our bodies, contributing to chronic inflammation - the leading cause of morbidity and mortality in Western societies.

We know that animals and animal products contain mostly "bad fat" (for example trans-fat and saturated fat) that is added to our own fat virtually unchanged - "lips to hips[308]".

We know that animals and animal products contain cholesterol, a compound that is made in sufficient quantities in our own bodies but dietary intake can directly lead to vascular disease, including heart failure and strokes[309].

Another substance analogous to cholesterol that we make in our own bodies, as do all animals, but do not want contributions from animals that we consume is arachidonic acid. Arachidonic acid is a key substrate for the synthesis of proinflammatory compounds that can adversely affect mental health via a cascade of neuroinflammation[310]. Studies have shown that relatively high amounts of arachidonic acid in our blood correlated positively with the severity of depression[311].

---

[308] I first saw this phrase written by Dr. Joel Fuhrman, who takes a similar stance to ours on the importance of nutrient density; Fuhrman, J. (2011). Eat to Live: The Amazing Nutrient-Rich Program for Fast and Sustained Weight Loss (Vol. Revised). Boston: Little, Brown and Company.

[309] Dr. Roberts, Editor and Chief of the American Journal of Cardiology, has been advocating cholesterol as the source of vascular disease in editorials for more than a decade, such as the following reference. Roberts, W. (2010). It's the Cholesterol, Stupid! *The American Journal of Cardiology, 106*(9), 1364-1366.

[310] Beezhold, B., Johnston, C., & Daigle, D. (2010). Vegetarian diets are associated with healthy mood states: A cross-sectional study in Seventh Day Adventist adults. *Nutr J Nutrition Journal, 9*, 26-26.

[311] Adams, P. B., Lawson, S., Sanigorski, A., & Sinclair, A. J. (1996). Arachidonic acid to eicosapentaenoic acid ratio in blood correlates posi-

Therefore, in our examination of macronutrient and micronutrient compositions, we shall not consider animals or animal products except as further illustrations of why they should not be part of a rational dietary pattern.

WATER

The only liquid I recommend consuming is water. Technically, the beverage water is not a whole-food varied-plant source, although much of our daily intake of water is from fruits and vegetables. Water is both a reactant in the light-dependent photosynthesis reaction and a product of the light-independent photosynthesis reaction, but overall, water must be provided exogenously to the plant, which retains a considerable amount of water for structure and chemical synthesis.

The best source of water is from non-contaminated spring water, originating from an underground water supply that flows upward to the earth's surface. The deeper the water source underground, the higher the mineral content. The original source of that water is usually rainwater, although deep sources of water conceivably could have been present with the formation of the earth[312].

One morning, as I was extracting the fat content of almonds that had soaked in water overnight to make almond "milk" for my oat bran, it came to mind that it was unnecessary to add a white colored liquid to my cereal. I had been conditioned since a young child to associate breakfast with cereal and cereal with "milk" or otherwise a fatty white fluid. My almond milk production threw out the most nutritious part of the almond,

---

tively with clinical symptoms of depression. Lipids, 31 (Suppl.), S157–S161.

[312] Cowen, Ron (9 May 2013). "Common source for Earth and Moon water". Nature. doi:10.1038/nature.2013.12963.

85% of the protein, 78% of the magnesium, and 75% of the fiber and loss of other nutrients. From that point forward, I use filtered tap water as my hydrating fluid, as on cereal; if I wish to add almonds, I just add whole or crushed almonds and get the whole-food nutrition.

Gronk and all his predecessors for millions of years drank from lakes and streams that primarily were generated from spring water (plus direct rainwater). Typical mineral content includes calcium, sodium, and magnesium. A less common metal present in some spring water is an ionic form of lithium.

MAGNESIUM

At the risk of sounding reductionist, there does appear to be an insufficient intake of magnesium by most Americans. The latest data indicates that 68% of Americans do not consume the recommended daily intake of magnesium (420 mg per day) and 19% of Americans do not consume even half the government's recommended daily intake of magnesium[313].

Would a serious whole-food varied-plant diet provide adequate magnesium? Maybe. But thinking of by-gone millennia in which greens were the food of choice (and spring water/ rain water the only beverage) does raise some doubts. As an example, consider spinach and oat bran, both considered good sources of magnesium.

A dose of 30 grams (one cup) of spinach has 23.7 mg of magnesium; 96 grams of oats (one and a half cups) has 96 mg of magnesium. But on a per calorie basis spinach has 3.4 mg

---

[313] King, D. E., Mainous, A. G., Geesey, M. E., & Woolson, R. F. (2005). Dietary Magnesium and C-reactive Protein Levels. *Journal of the American College of Nutrition, 24*(3), 166-171. doi:10.1080/ 07315724. 2005.10719461.

magnesium compared to 0.45 mg for oats. On a per dry weight comparison spinach has 3.4 mg/g of magnesium compared to 1.7 mg/g for oats. That's more than five times the magnesium content in spinach compared to oats.

Magnesium, one of the most essential minerals in the human body, is a co-factor in more than 600 known enzymatic reactions[314]. Magnesium is widely connected with brain biochemistry and, as a result, a deficiency is associated with a variety of neuromuscular and psychiatric symptoms such as depression, psychosis, agitation and irritability, headaches, seizures, muscular weakness, anxiety, insomnia, fatigue, confusion and cognitive changes; this is reversible with restoration of sufficient magnesium levels[315].

The diets of those clinically depressed is correlated with low intake of magnesium; research indicates an inverse relationship between dietary magnesium content and depressive symptoms[316]. Suicidal depression particularly appears to be related to magnesium insufficiency; for example[317], data

---

[314] Kantak, K. M. (1988). Magnesium deficiency alters aggressive behavior and catecholamine function. *Behavioral Neuroscience, 102*(2), 304-311. doi:10.1037//0735-7044.102.2.304.

[315] Papadopol V, Tuchendria E, Palamaru I: Magnesium and some psychological features in two groups of pupils (magnesium and psychic features) (2001). Magnes Res, 14, 27–32.

[316] Jacka, F. N., Overland, S., Stewart, R., Tell, G. S., Bjelland, I., & Mykletun, A. (2009). Association between magnesium intake and depression and anxiety in community-dwelling adults: The Hordaland Health Study. *Australian and New Zealand Journal of Psychiatry, 43*(1), 45-52. doi:10.1080/00048670802534408.

[317] Banki, C. M., Arató, M., & Kilts, C. D. (1986). Aminergic Studies and Cerebrospinal Fluid Cations in Suicide. *Ann NY Acad Sci Annals of the New York Academy of Sciences, 487*(1 Psychobiology), 221-230. doi:10.1111/j.1749-6632.1986.tb27901.x.

indicate that magnesium concentration in cerebrospinal fluid was low in patients with history of suicidal behavior[318].

The take-home here is to *eat your greens*. A magnesium level may be useful as an initial clinical workup for psychiatric symptoms. If your magnesium level is verified to be low and there are accompanying psychiatric symptoms, your provider may choose to add a supplement of 600 – 800 mg per day of any of the various forms of magnesium available (except magnesium oxide, which is not bioavailable).

LITHIUM

Lithium was once used as a key ingredient in a soft drink invented in 1929 by Charles Leipe Grigg, an American from Price Branch, Missouri. He initially called his drink "Bib-Label Lithiated Lemon-Lime Sodas". He later changed the name to " 7 Up Lithiated Lemon-Lime".

The "7" in the name comes from the atomic mass of lithium. He called his drink 7-Up presumably because of the ability of lithium to elevate the mood. These were obviously low concentrations of lithium citrate; as in deep warm springs yielding lithium salts that have been used for centuries to calm visitors at spas.

In 1962, George Winokur[319] introduced lithium to Washington University in St. Louis (where I happened to do my adult

---

[318] Banki, C. M., Vojnik, M., Papp, Z., Balla, K. Z., & Arató, M. (1985). Cerebrospinal fluid magnesium and calcium related to amine metabolites, diagnosis, and suicide attempts. *Biological Psychiatry, 20*(2), 163-171. doi:10.1016/0006-3223(85)90076-9.

[319] Dr. Winokur, together with colleagues Eli Robbins and Samuel Guze — with whom I studied while at Washington University — established the first written formalized criteria for mental disorders, the so-called Feighner criteria, establishing the basic model for the Diagnostic

psychiatric residency and child fellowship), having the Barnes Hospital pharmacy make up the pills and achieving an "amazing remission" in a patient who had failed on thorazine treatment and eighteen sessions of electroconvulsive therapy. This was the beginning of the widespread use of lithium in the United States for bipolar disorder and later for mania prophylaxis and still later as an adjunctive treatment for depression; it is today the only psychotropic medication that does not carry the "black box" disclaimer of potentially leading to suicidal thoughts.

The lithium ion is the third element on the periodic table and as it is just above sodium, it does have similar chemical properties to sodium. In the beginning of the twentieth century, lithium salt was prescribed as a substitute for table salt because it was not associated with high blood pressure; however, use in high arbitrary doses could lead to toxicity, so was discontinued for that purpose.

Lithium appears to be a nutritionally essential trace element found predominantly in plant-derived foods and drinking water[320], although its function has not been fully described. This trace element is typically present in all human organs and tissues, and is equally distributed in body water, as lithium is absorbed from the intestinal tract and excreted by the kidneys.

---

and Statistical Manual series (DSM). The motivation for these criteria was totally as a way to compare research studies on similar patients and not to be taken too literally, a position lost in the many later DSM versions and now falling in disrepute. Dr. Winokur is credited with the statement "Making up new sets of diagnostic criteria in American psychiatry has become a cottage industry with little attempt at quality control", source Glicksman, A. (2009). "Jesus Loves Me, that I Know, for the Chi-Square Tells Me So" Privileged and Non-Privileged Approaches to the Study of Religion and Aging: A Response. *Journal of Religion, Spirituality & Aging, 21*(4), 316-317. doi:10.1080/15528030903127155.

[320] Schrauzer GN (2002) Lithium: occurrence, dietary intakes, nutritional essentiality. J Am Coll Nutr 21:14–21.

Recent research studies measuring the effects of trace levels of lithium, commonly found in lithia waters (on the order of 2 mg/liter compared to typical pharmacologic doses of 900 mg/day), have demonstrated neuroprotective abilities[321] as well as improvements in mood and cognitive function[322].

Studies on the local concentration of lithium in some municipal water supplies suggest that lithium has moderating effects on suicidal and violent criminal behaviors[323].

DEHYDRATION

Severe dehydration results in acute confusion, delirium, organ failure and potentially death. But even mild levels of dehydration (1%) result in increased headaches and difficulty concentrating[324]. Assurance of adequate hydration requires conscious supplementation, regardless of a thirst motivator.

In addition to a whole-food varied-plant diet, four 12 ounce glasses of water is recommended. I keep a paper cup dispenser

---

[321] Xu, J., Culman, J., Blume, A., Brecht, S., & Gohlke, P. (2003). Chronic Treatment With a Low Dose of Lithium Protects the Brain Against Ischemic Injury by Reducing Apoptotic Death. *Stroke, 34*(5), 1287-1292. doi:10.1161/01.str.0000066308.25088.64.

[322] Schrauzer, De Vroey. *Effects of Nutritional Lithium Supplementation on Mood.* Biological Trace Element Research Volume 40 1994 pages 89-101.

[323] Schrauzer, G. N., & Shrestha, K. P. (1990). Lithium in drinking water and the incidences of crimes, suicides, and arrests related to drug addictions. *Biological Trace Element Research, 25*(2), 105-113. doi:10.1007/bf02990271

[324] Armstrong, L. E., Ganio, M. S., Casa, D. J., Lee, E. C., Mcdermott, B. P., Klau, J. F., . . . Lieberman, H. R. (2011). Mild Dehydration Affects Mood in Healthy Young Women. *Journal of Nutrition, 142*(2), 382-388. doi:10.3945/jn.111.142000.

near every source of water in my home and drink a five-ounce cup or two each time I wash my hands.

MACRONUTRIENTS

We shall begin our exploration of the optimal food for health and happiness, or in other words physical and cognitive/emotional wellness, by examining the overall need for energy. This is the prime function of the macronutrients.

> *We have evolved genetically to depend on plants; conversely, there are a number of reasons why consumption of animal and animal products is dangerous to our body and minds.*

CHAPTER 9

Fat

"The act of putting into your mouth what the earth has grown is perhaps your most direct interaction with the earth."

Frances Moore Lappé

YOUR FAT

The human brain is an organ that is 60% fat by dry weight, an organ which functions through structural and metabolic utilization of fats, including essential fatty acids (EFAs), cholesterol, and other naturally occurring fatty substances called lipids.

Fat is one of the three main sources of energy, including carbohydrates and protein, known as macronutrients. Macronutrients are hydrocarbon sources that are plentiful on earth because of the ability of plants to manufacture them through photosynthesis.

When we talk about fats in the body we are generally referring to fatty acids, the building blocks for fat in a fashion similar to how amino acids make up proteins. Amino acids can be combined to produce different proteins, and fatty acids can be joined together to create different kinds of fat.

Fats are vital to cell function. They are also required for digestion, absorption, and transportation of fat soluble nutrients such as carotenoids (more generally terpenoids), and vitamins A, D, E, and K.

Fats are also known as triglycerides because there are three fatty acid chains connected by a central core molecular arrangement; triglycerides comprise about 98% of our dietary fat intake[325]. The chains are made up of carbon molecules with hydrogen attachments, thus the term hydrocarbons. Many human cells can use either glucose or fatty acids for fuel but use of glucose is highly more efficient.

OMEGA-3 FATTY ACIDS

Omega-3 fatty acids are *polyunsaturated fatty acids* (PUFAs) - hydrocarbon chains with one end labeled *alpha* and the other end *omega*. The "poly" in polyunsaturated means "many" and unsaturated means there are *double* carbon bonds, so taken together these fatty acids have many carbon double bonds. The "3" in omega-3 refers to the first double bond from the omega end occurring at the third carbon.

That's all unnecessary for you to know, but this molecule is so important, as you shall see, that the name should be a little more real to you now.

---

[325] Otten, J. J., Hellwig, J. P., & Meyers, L. D. (Eds.). (2006). *Dietary reference intakes: the essential guide to nutrient requirements.* National Academies Press, p.123.

There are three types of omega-3 fatty acids:

- α-linolenic acid (ALA)
- eicosapentaenoic acid (EPA)
- docosahexaenoic acid (DHA)

To assure adequate daily omega-3 ALA intake, eat one tablespoon of flaxseeds per day. They need to be crushed, for example in a coffee grinder.

Of these three, only ALA is *essential* because it can lead to synthesis of EPA and subsequently to DHA. ALA is manufactured by *all* plants and is the most abundant fat on the planet, likely having a regulatory function in chloroplasts[326]; it has a high concentration in seeds, such as flaxseeds and chia seeds. ALA, a short-chain omega-3 fatty acid, can then elongate into the long-chain fatty acids EPA and DHA; there does not need to be any dietary intake at all of EPA and DHA if there is adequate consumption of ALA[327]. That is a critical point to remember.

An *adequate intake*[328] (AI) for ALA is 1.6 grams/day for men and 1.1 grams/day for women[329], or about 0.6 – 1.2 percent of

---

[326] Vannice, G., & Rasmussen, H. (2014). Position of the Academy of Nutrition and Dietetics: Dietary Fatty Acids for Healthy Adults. *Journal of the Academy of Nutrition and Dietetics, 114*(1), 136-153. doi:10.1016/j.jand.2013.11.001.

[327] Domenichiello, A. F., Kitson, A. P., & Bazinet, R. P. (2015). Is docosahexaenoic acid synthesis from α-linolenic acid sufficient to supply the adult brain? *Progress in Lipid Research, 59*, 54-66. doi:10.1016/j.plipres.2015.04.002.

[328] *Adequate Intake* for individual nutrients is similar to *Recommended Dietary Allowances* but less certain.

total caloric intake per day[330]. This can be obtained with a whole-food varied-plant diet. To *assure* adequate intake, consider using one or more tablespoons of flaxseeds daily (be certain to crush or grind these little hard-shelled seeds or they could pass through the GI system undigested).

THE BAD FATS: FISH OIL SUPPLEMENTS?

Fish oil supplements have been popularized as an omega-3 option. However, the omega-3s found in fish oils (EPA and DHA) are actually highly unstable molecules that tend to decompose and unleash dangerous free radicals, making these supplements an unfavorable option. In addition, current research demonstrates that taking fish oil supplements does not actually produce significant protection of vascular health[331]. And such supplements, being processed and non-whole food extracts from fish livers, introduce the unknowns of what additional oils and potential toxins are present.

What about the treatment of existing clinical depression with EPA or DHA supplements? Numerous studies have shown neither was superior to placebo for the treatment of depression[332].

---

[329] Food and Nutrition Board. (2005). *Dietary reference intakes for energy, carbohydrate, fiber, fat, fatty acids, cholesterol, protein, and amino acids* (p. 423). Washington, D.C.: National Academies Press.

[330] Otten, J. J., Hellwig, J. P., & Meyers, L. D. (Eds.). (2006). *Dietary reference intakes: the essential guide to nutrient requirements*. National Academies Press.

[331] Kwak, S., Myung, S., & Lee, Y. (2012). Efficacy of omega-3 fatty acid supplements (eicosapentaenoic acid and docosahexaenoic acid) in the secondary prevention of cardiovascular disease: A meta-analysis of randomized, double-blind, placebo- controlled trials. *Archives of Internal Medicine Arch Intern Med, 172,* 986-994.

[332] Mischoulon, D., Nierenberg, A. A., Schettler, P. J., Kinkead, B. L., Fehling, K., Martinson, M. A., & Rapaport, M. H. (2014). A Double-Blind, Randomized Controlled Clinical Trial Comparing Eicosapentaenoic Acid

> *You need adequate intake of the essential omega-3s, in proper balance with omega-6. You do not need to eat fish or take EPA/ DHA supplements. ALA alone can provide these requirements.*

A meta-analysis of all trials of EPA/ DHA supplementation indicated no significant benefit compared with placebo; the studies indicating positive treatment efficacy in the published literature was thought to be publication bias, that is, studies showing no benefit tended not to get published at all compared to those with some positive effects.

Research has shown that omega-3s are found in a more stable form, ALA, in vegetables, fruits, and beans.[333] In fact, according to a European Prospective Investigation into Cancer and Nutrition, women on vegan diets actually have more EPA and DHA in their blood compared to fish-eaters, meat-eaters, and lacto-ovo vegetarians[334].

NO FISH STORY

Eating fish is problematic from a number of standpoints. Farm-raised fish often does not contain EPA and DHA because the

---

Versus Docosahexaenoic Acid for Depression. *J. Clin. Psychiatry The Journal of Clinical Psychiatry,* 54-61. doi:10.4088/jcp.14m08986.

[333] Odeleye, O., & Watson, R. (1991). Health implications of the n-3 fatty acids. *American Journal of Clinical Nutrition, 53,* 177-178.

[334] Welch, A., Shakya-Shrestha, S., Lentjes, M., Wareham, N., & Khaw, K. (2010). Dietary intake and status of n-3 polyunsaturated fatty acids in a population of fish-eating and non-fish-eating meat-eaters, vegetarians, and vegans and the precursor-product ratio of linolenic acid to long-chain n-3 polyunsaturated fatty acids: Results. *American Journal of Clinical Nutrition, 92,* 1040-1051.

source of these omega-3s is actually algae that are typically not available for farm-raised fish. Wild-caught fish, on the other hand, may contain various toxic substances such as persistent organic pollutants (POPs), including dioxins, polychlorinated biphenyls (PCBs), organochlorine pesticides, and polybrominated diphenyl ethers as well as heavy metals, including mercury, lead, and cadmium – all adversely affecting human health[335].

Toxins may be responsible for the finding of a significant increase in risk of atrial fibrillation – an irregular heartbeat rhythm associated with stroke and dementia[336]. Even antidepressants such as Prozac have been found to bioaccumulate in fish, presumably from unused product excreted in human urine finding its way into water supplies – but the quantities of pharmaceutics like Prozac are well below being clinically useful – and are located primarily in fish brains[337].

A meta-analysis of prospective studies of fish consumption concluded[338]:

---

[335] Jacobs, D. R., Ruzzin, J., & Lee, D. (2014). Environmental pollutants: Downgrading the fish food stock affects chronic disease risk. *J Intern Med Journal of Internal Medicine, 276*(3), 240-242. doi:10.1111/joim.12205.

[336] Shen, J., Johnson, V. M., Sullivan, L. M., Jacques, P. F., Magnani, J. W., Lubitz, S. A., . . . Benjamin, E. J. (2010). Dietary factors and incident atrial fibrillation: The Framingham Heart Study. *American Journal of Clinical Nutrition, 93*(2), 261-266. doi:10.3945/ajcn.110.001305.

[337] Ramirez, A. J., Brain, R. A., Usenko, S., Mottaleb, M. A., O'donnell, J. G., Stahl, L. L., . . . Chambliss, C. K. (2009). Occurrence Of Pharmaceuticals And Personal Care Products In Fish: Results Of A National Pilot Study In The United States.*Environmental Toxicology and Chemistry Environ Toxicol Chem, 28*(12), 2587. doi:10.1897/08-561.1.

[338] Ruzzin, J., & Jacobs, D. R. (2012). The secret story of fish: Decreasing nutritional value due to pollution? *British Journal of Nutrition Br J Nutr, 108*(03), 397-399. doi:10.1017/s0007114512002048.

"These findings emphasize the background levels of POP, ... can completely counteract the potential benefits of omega-3 fatty acids and other nutrients present in fish ..."

One large longitudinal study of over 100,000 Japanese men and women were followed for up to 10 years; higher intakes of fish, with attendant increase in serum levels of EPA and DHA were not associated with a lower risk of suicide[339]. In fact, they found a significantly increased risk of suicide with high seafood omega-3 PUFA intake.

A similar result was found in a prospective study of over 10,000 Spanish participants on a Mediterranean dietary pattern[340]. High baseline fish consumption together with an increase in consumption was associated with an increased risk of mental disorders. But in the Mediterranean diet, it was the fruit, nuts, legumes and ratio of monounsaturated fats to saturated fats that was associated with good mental health, not the fish.

Another prospective cohort study performed with about 8,000 participants led the researchers to conclude[341]:

---

[339] Poudel-Tandukar, K., Nanri, A., Iwasaki, M., Mizoue, T., Matsushita, Y., Takahashi, Y., . . . Tsugane, S. (2011). Long chain n-3 fatty acids intake, fish consumption and suicide in a cohort of Japanese men and women — The Japan Public Health Center-based (JPHC) Prospective Study. *Journal of Affective Disorders, 129*(1-3), 282-288. doi:10.1016/j.jad.2010.07.014.

[340] Sánchez-Villegas, A., Delgado-Rodríguez, M., Alonso, A., Schlatter, J., Lahortiga, F., Majem, L. S., & Martínez-González, M. A. (2009). Association of the Mediterranean Dietary Pattern With the Incidence of Depression. *Arch Gen Psychiatry Archives of General Psychiatry, 66*(10), 1090. doi:10.1001/archgenpsychiatry.2009.129.

[341] Sanchez-Villegas, A., Henríquez, P., Figueiras, A., Ortuño, F., Lahortiga, F., & Martínez-González, M. A. (2007). Long chain omega-3 fatty

> *"Unexpectantly, when baseline and follow-up fish consumption were jointly considered in our analysis, a high baseline consumption together with an increment in consumption were associated with an increased risk of mental disorders."*

The reason for this was not understood but there was speculation that perhaps mercury compounds could be implicated.

The large Harvard cohort study of more than 200,000 US men and women followed for up to 22 years did not find evidence that intake of fish or DHA/ EPA supplements lowered the risk of completed suicides; in fact the trend was toward higher risks of suicide mortality[342].

DHA

Docosahexaenoic acid is highly concentrated in the brain, and is important for brain function in part by regulation of cell survival and neuroinflammation[343] [344]. DHA is the main omega-3 PUFA

---

acids intake, fish consumption and mental disorders in the SUN cohort study. *European Journal of Nutrition Eur J Nutr, 46*(6), 337-346. doi:10.1007/s00394-007-0671-x.

[342] Tsai, A. C., Lucas, M., Okereke, O. I., O'reilly, E. J., Mirzaei, F., Kawachi, I., . . . Willett, W. C. (2014). Suicide Mortality in Relation to Dietary Intake of n-3 and n-6 Polyunsaturated Fatty Acids and Fish: Equivocal Findings From 3 Large US Cohort Studies. *American Journal of Epidemiology, 179*(12), 1458-1466. doi:10.1093/aje/kwu086.

[343] Orr, S. K., Palumbo, S., Bosetti, F., Mount, H. T., Kang, J. X., Greenwood, C. E., . . . Bazinet, R. P. (2013). Unesterified docosahexaenoic acid is protective in neuroinflammation. *J. Neurochem. Journal of Neurochemistry, 127*(3), 378-393. doi:10.1111/jnc.12392.

in the brain as it is present at levels of about 10–15% of brain fatty acids, at least 50-times more than EPA and 200-times more than ALA[345]. DHA brain deficiencies are associated with cognitive deficits and anxiety[346]. Lower brain DHA concentration is present in major depressive disorder relative to controls[347].

DHA can cross the blood-brain-barrier, possibly by passive diffusion[348]. Therefore, dietary ALA in sufficient quantities can provide brain DHA synthesized in the liver. DHA synthesis from ALA is sufficient to maintain brain function; consumption of fish or fish oil is unnecessary[349], as previously emphasized.

---

[344] Lukiw, W. J. (2005). A role for docosahexaenoic acid-derived neuroprotectin D1 in neural cell survival and Alzheimer disease. *Journal of Clinical Investigation,115*(10), 2774-2783. doi:10.1172/jci25420.

[345] Igarashi, M., Ma, K., Gao, F., Kim, H., Greenstein, D., Rapoport, S. I., & Rao, J. S. (2010). Brain lipid concentrations in bipolar disorder. *Journal of Psychiatric Research, 44*(3), 177-182. doi:10.1016/j.jpsychires. 2009.08.001.

[346] Brenna, J. T. (2011). Animal studies of the functional consequences of suboptimal polyunsaturated fatty acid status during pregnancy, lactation and early post-natal life. *Maternal & Child Nutrition, 7*, 59-79. doi:10.1111/j.1740-8709.2011.00301.x.

[347] Mcnamara, R. K., Hahn, C., Jandacek, R., Rider, T., Tso, P., Stanford, K. E., & Richtand, N. M. (2007). Selective Deficits in the Omega-3 Fatty Acid Docosahexaenoic Acid in the Postmortem Orbitofrontal Cortex of Patients with Major Depressive Disorder. *Biological Psychiatry, 62*(1), 17-24. doi:10.1016/j.biopsych.2006.08.026.

[348] Ouellet, M., Emond, V., Chen, C. T., Julien, C., Bourasset, F., Oddo, S., . . . Calon, F. (2009). Diffusion of docosahexaenoic and eicosapentaenoic acids through the blood–brain barrier: An in situ cerebral perfusion study. *Neurochemistry International, 55*(7), 476-482. doi:10.1016/j.neuint.2009.04.018.

[349] Domenichiello, A. F., Kitson, A. P., & Bazinet, R. P. (2015). Is docosahexaenoic acid synthesis from α-linolenic acid sufficient to supply the adult brain? *Progress in Lipid Research, 59*, 54-66. doi:10.1016/j.plipres.2015.04.002.

> *Dietary ALA, as present, for example, in flaxseeds, can provide the other essential fatty acids EPA and DHA; EPA and DHA do not need to be consumed.*

POSSIBLE MECHANISMS OF OMEGA-3 PUFAS IN PREVENTING AND REVERSING DEPRESSION

Several mechanisms have been proposed to explain the link between omega-3 PUFAs and mental wellness. Omega-3 PUFAs are well documented inhibitors of both pro-inflammatory cytokines so that one mechanism of the protective effect could be as anti-inflammatory agents[350]. Another possible explanation is the importance of omega-3 PUFAs in maintaining membrane integrity and fluidity, which is crucial for neurotransmitter binding[351]. Furthermore, omega-3 PUFAs affect brain-derived neurotropic factor (BDNF), which encourages synaptic plasticity, provides neuroprotection, and enhances neuro-transmission and associated antidepressant effects[352].

---

[350] Kiecolt-Glaser, J. K., Belury, M. A., Porter, K. Beversdorf, D. Q., Lemeshow, S., and Glaser, R. (2007). Depressive symptoms, omega-6:omega-3 fatty acids, and inflammation in older adults. Psychosomatic medicine 69: 217-224.

[351] Su, K. P. (2009). Biological mechanism of antidepressant effect of omega-3 fatty acids: how does fish oil act as a 'mind-body interface'? Neurosignals, 17, 144-152.

[352] Logan, A. C. (2003). Neurobehavioral aspects of omega-3 fatty acids: possible mechanisms and therapeutic value in major depression. Altern Med Rev 8: 410-425.

BUILDING A HAPPIER BRAIN: NEUROGENESIS

Only quite recently has it become apparent that there is growth of new neurons throughout our lifespan, so called neurogenesis. This is restricted to only a few brain regions, such as the hippocampus[353], but the neurogenesis taking place there has implications for learning and memory[354] and psychiatric disorders such as schizophrenia[355] and clinical depression.

Omega-3 fatty acids enhance adult hippocampal neurogenesis associated with cognitive and emotional/ behavioral processes, promoting synaptic plasticity[356], yet another mechanism for mood improvement from these compounds.

OMEGA-6 TO OMEGA-3 RATIO "6-TO-3"

Omega-6s are pro-inflammatory, while omega-3s have an anti-inflammatory effect, but it's not only the amounts of these fatty acids that are important but also their balance, that is the omega-6 to omega-3 ratio, the "6-to-3" ratio.

---

[353] Kempermann G, Jessberger S, Steiner B, Kronenberg G (2004) Milestones of neuronal development in the adult hippocampus. Trends Neurosci 27:447–452.

[354] Deng W, Aimone JB, Gage FH (2010) New neurons and new memories: how does adult hippocampal neurogenesis affect learning and memory? Nat Rev Neurosci 11:339–350.

[355] Ouchi Y, Banno Y, Shimizu Y, Ando S, Hasegawa H, Adachi K, Iwamoto T (2013) Reduced adult hippocampal neurogenesis and working memory deficits in the Dgcr8-deficient mouse model of 22q11.2 deletion-associated schizophrenia can be rescued by IGF2. J Neurosci 33:9408–9419.

[356] Crupi, R., Marino, A., & Cuzzocrea, S. (2013). N-3 Fatty Acids: Role in Neurogenesis and Neuroplasticity. CMC Current Medicinal Chemistry, 20(24), 2953-2963. doi:10.2174/09298673113209990140.

Our genetics evolved on a diet with a 6-to-3 of about 1:1 whereas in Western diets the ratio is about 20:1[357].

Modern refining and processing of foods as well as cultural dietary selections, particularly in industrialized nations, have also led to the increase in the consumption of omega-6 PUFAs and a relative deficiency of omega-3 PUFAs[358]. Correlated with this dramatic decline in the consumption of omega-3s is the rapidly rising prevalence of mood disorders[359]. A number of studies are now suggesting that this change in fatty acid intake is associated with the development of depression and the increase in suicidal tendency in those previously diagnosed with depression[360].

High 6-to-3 ratios promotes the pathogenesis of vascular disease, cancer, and inflammatory and autoimmune diseases, whereas lower ratios exert suppressive effects.[361] For example, in the secondary prevention of cardiovascular disease, a ratio of even 4:1 was associated with a 70% decrease in total mortality[362].

---

[357] Mazza, M., Pomponi, M., Janiri, L., Bria, P. and Mazza, S. (2006). Omega 3 Fatty Acids and Antioxidants in Neurological and Psychiatric Disease: An Overview. Progress in Neuropsychopharmacology and Biological Psychiatry, 31: 12-26.

[358] Young, C. and Martin, A. 2003. Omega-3 fatty acids in mood disorders: an overview. Rev Bras Psiquiatr, 25, 184-187.

[359] Sublette, M. E., Hibbeln, J. R., Galfalvey, H., Oquendo, M. A., and Mann, J. J. (2006). Omega-3 polyunsaturated essential fatty acid status as a predictor of future suicide risk. Am J Psychiatry, 163, 1100-1102.

[360] ibid.

[361] Simopoulos, A. (2002). The importance of the ratio of omega-6 to omega-3 essential fatty acids. *Biomedicine & Pharmacotherapy, 56*(8), 365-379.

[362] ibid.

---

*A distorted ratio of omega-6 to omega-3 may
be one of the most damaging aspects of the
Western diet.*

FAT COMPOSITION

There is conflicting information on the amount of total fat that
is optimal in our diets. The generally accepted reference
*Dietary reference intakes: the essential guide to nutrient
requirements* of the National Academies Press suggests energy
intake for fat and carbohydrates while holding protein intake at
no less than 10% of total energy intake[363].

Neither an Estimated Average Requirement (EAR), and thus a
Recommended Dietary Allowance (RDA), nor an Adequate
Intake (AI) was set for total fat

> *"because data were insufficient to determine a
> defined intake level at which risk of inadequacy
> or prevention of chronic disease occurs."*

An *Acceptable Macro-nutrient Distribution Range* (AMDR) has
been estimated for total fat at 20–35 percent of energy for
adults[364]. However, this is based on

---

[363] Food and Nutrition Board. (2005). *Dietary reference intakes for
energy, carbohydrate, fiber, fat, fatty acids, cholesterol, protein, and
amino acids* (p. 423). Washington, D.C.: National Academies Press.

[364] Otten, J. J., Hellwig, J. P., & Meyers, L. D. (Eds.). (2006). *Dietary
reference intakes: the essential guide to nutrient requirements*. National
Academies Press, p. 70.

> *"main food sources of total fat are butter, margarine, vegetable oils, visible fat on meat and poultry products, whole milk, egg yolk, nuts, and baked goods, such as cookies, doughnuts, pastries and cakes and various fried foods[365]."*

Note that every item in this list, except nuts, is non whole-food varied plants; it is processed or animal-based.

It appears that the Standard American Diet (SAD) is accepted by the dietary guidelines to establish an "acceptable" range of daily caloric fat consumption. However, there is no "acceptable" rationale for such a high fat reference range. Cholesterol, trans-fat, saturated fatty acid intake are suggested to be "as low as possible", rather than zero. "Added sugar" is suggested to be no more than 25% by calories, rather than zero.

Every study referenced in this book on the basis of general health, and mental health in particular, recommends a whole-food varied-plant diet, rather than a diet based on animals or processed foods.

Therefore, we shall suggest here actual, healthy recommendations for macronutrients.

A clue to a reasonable percentage of caloric contribution from fat is revealed by examining the fat content of typical fruits and vegetables such as those in the following table[366].

---

[365] Ibid, p. 123.

[366] USDA's National Nutrient Database for Standard Reference; Foods List. (n.d.). Retrieved August 20, 2016, from https://ndb.nal.usda.gov/ndb/foods.

Fat

You may be surprised that all fruits and vegetables have a significant fat content, but only nuts and seeds have a high fat content. A whole-food varied-plant diet with a modicum of nuts and seeds would have about 10% fat. We shall take that number (10%) as a "reasonable" estimate of percent caloric fat for a healthy diet, as seen in the table for kale, broccoli, whole wheat bread, and tomatoes.

Figure 6 Fat, Omega-3, Omega-6 and "6 to 3" ratios

Food	% fat	omega 3/g	omega 6/g	omega 6/3
flaxseeds	66.1	0.24520	0.06354	0.3
kale, raw	11.8	0.01163	0.00888	0.8
broccoli, raw	9.0	0.00201	0.00160	0.8
black beans	3.4	0.00307	0.00368	1.2
banana raw	3.1	0.00109	0.00184	1.7
walnuts	83.5	0.09468	0.39721	4.2
apple, raw	2.8	0.00062	0.00299	4.8
pasta, whole wheat	6.6	0.00176	0.01449	8.2
sweet potato, raw	0.5	0.00004	0.00058	13.3
bread, whole wheat	12.2	0.00041	0.00936	23.0
tomato, raw	9.4	0.00054	0.01440	26.7

Also shown on the table is the total weight in grams of omega-6 PUFA and omega-6 PUFA per dry total weight (also in grams) of each food listed. Flaxseeds have an extraordinarily favorable content of these nutrients; for example, one tablespoon of whole flax seeds weighs about 10 grams of which 0.7 grams is water, so multiplying the numbers under the omega-6/g and omega-3/g columns gives:

Total amount of omega-3 = (10.0 − 0.7) X 0.24520 = 2.3 grams and

Total amount of omega-6 = (10.0 − 0.7) X 0.06354 = 0.6 grams

Recalling the AI (adequate intake) for omega-3 (1.6 grams/day for men and 1.1 grams/day for women), this single tablespoon of flaxseeds is sufficient for the day.

Legumes are acceptable sources for these essential fats: a cup of black beans contains 0.5 grams of omega-3; as are nuts: four English walnuts contains 1.4 grams of omega-3.

Note, too, in the table the ratios of omega-6 to omega-3. For vegetables this ratio is near to 1:1, the ratio experienced by our primate ancestors; while the ratio is higher for grains and fruits, but the total amount of omega-3 and omega-6 is low.

HOW TO ACHIEVE AN ADEQUATE OMEGA-3 INTAKE AND 6-TO-3 RATIO

Among modern societies, the Japanese consume the most fish, typically about 3 ounces daily[367]. The most commonly consumed fish in Japan is Pacific mackerel; 3 ounces would contain about 1.4 g of omega-3, still less than the AI of 1.6 g/day for a typical male, according to the aforementioned Food and Nutrition Board of the National Academia of Sciences[368]. The Standard American Diet (SAD) has at most one meal of fish per week. Just taking the same figure of 3 ounces per day of mackerel that would be the equivalent of 0.2 g/ day, well under

---

[367] Sekikawa, A., Curb, J. D., Ueshima, H., El-Saed, A., Kadowaki, T., Abbott, R. D., . . . Kuller, L. H. (2008). Marine-Derived n-3 Fatty Acids and Atherosclerosis in Japanese, Japanese-American, and White Men. Journal of the American College of Cardiology, 52(6), 417-424. doi:10.1016/j.jacc.2008.03.047.

368 Dietary reference intakes for energy, carbohydrate, fiber, fat, fatty acids, cholesterol, protein, and amino acids. (2005). Washington, D.C.: National Academies Press.

the AI, and not being a daily dose but an average, it is not necessarily stored in the body and used as needed.

So something is fishy. Even an advanced society that bases its dietary pattern on fish may not be getting an adequate intake of omega-3. How can this be?

The answer is revealed through evolution. For 85 million years as primates our dietary pattern was that of whole-food varied-plants; although the specific composition of this diet changed over time and location, there was undoubtedly a substantial contribution from green leafy plants.

An engineering-type of estimation of what this might mean in terms of omega-3 consumption follows. Consider contemporary common kale. One hundred grams of kale contains about 180 mg of omega-3 fatty acids and 138 mg of omega-6 for a favorable 6-to-3 ratio of about 0.8. How much kale would one have to eat to get 1.6 grams of omega-3, AI for males and females today?

Crunching the numbers gives 888 grams of kale or almost two pounds. That's about ten cups of chopped kale.

My own best attempt to maximize intake of kale in a smoothie using a high-speed blender peaked at about 5 cups but that was limited primarily by my kale cache. It is possible, of course, to eat two pounds of kale but not particularly pleasant or necessary in today's society.

Did our ancestors eat that many leafy greens? Two pounds of kale equals only about 440 calories so either they ate a lot more leafy greens than that, or they supplemented with a variety of other energy-dense foods. Likely both. So the reason we need to have a higher intake of omega-3s appears to be that it's inconvenient these days to eat anywhere near the amount of leafy greens that we evolved to eat. Besides, the bitter factor leads us to more "tasty" energy-dense cuisine.

> *The reason why our diets are low in omega 3 is that we are eating much less leafy green type vegetables than our distant ancestors*

CHAPTER 10

Protein

"If one tells the truth, one is sure, sooner or later, to be found out."

Oscar Wilde

PROTEIN IN PERSPECTIVE

Each neurotransmitter in the brain is made from specific amino acids through a series of chemical reactions. For example, the neurotransmitter dopamine is made from the amino acid tyrosine and the neurotransmitter serotonin is made from tryptophan. A sufficient supply of these amino acids is critical for necessary neurotransmitter levels and functioning in the brain. It has been known for decades that insufficient amounts of certain neurotransmitters is associated with mental illness – low levels of the neurotransmitter serotonin with clinical depression (the so-called monoamine theory of depression); disturbed levels of the neurotransmitter dopamine with schizophrenia, norepinephrine with bipolar disorder, acetylcholine with dementia.

These neurotransmitters cannot cross the blood-brain barrier and therefore need the necessary chemical reactants, including amino acids, to cross the barrier for synthesis in the brain.

Just as an interesting side note, the fact that these critical human neurotransmitters cannot cross the blood-brain barrier is unfortunate because they are present in plants. Pineapples, bananas, kiwis, plums, and tomatoes contain serotonin[369]; high concentrations of dopamine and norepinephrine have been found in avocados, tomatoes, eggplants, spinach, and peas[370]; acetylcholine has been found in many species of plants as well as in bacteria and fungi[371]. Of course, as plants do not have a known nervous system, the functions of these compounds are different, ranging from germination to flowering.

> *Plants synthesize all amino acids, including the essential amino acids that mammals are unable to make.*

Both animal and plant proteins are made up of about twenty common amino acids. The proportion of these amino acids

---

[369] Gharibzadeh, S., Hosseini, M., Shoar, S., & Hoseini, S. S. (2010). Depression and Fruit Treatment. *Journal of Neuropsychiatry, 22*(4). doi:10.1176/appi.neuropsych.22.4.451-m.e25.

[370] Feldman, J. M., E. M. Lee, C. A. Castleberry, 1987. Catecholamine and serotonin content of foods: effect on urinary excretion of homovanillic and 5-hydroxyindoleacetic acid. J. Am. Diet. Assoc., 87, 1031–1035.

[371] Tretyn, A., R. E. Kendrick, 1991. Acetylcholine in plants: presence, metabolism and mechanism of action. Bot. Rev., 57, 33–73.

varies as a characteristic of a given protein, but all food proteins contain some of each.

Plants easily make hydrocarbons; the "hydro" source is hydrogen from the water molecule (literally called di-hydro-oxygen) and the source of carbon is carbon dioxide in the air combined with water in photosynthesis to produce a wide variety of hydrocarbons. However, amino acids contain a substantial quantity of the element nitrogen obtained by plants from the soil and not as readily available nor as easily assimilated as hydrogen or carbon.

Nine amino acids—histidine, isoleucine, leucine, lysine, methionine, phenylalanine, threonine, tryptophan, and valine—are not synthesized by mammals and are therefore essential or indispensable nutrients. These are commonly called the *essential amino acids (EAA)* and they are of plant origin.

HOW MUCH PROTEIN?

Human protein requirements and recommended protein intake have been investigated primarily through the so-called *nitrogen balance* technique, which in simple terms measures the level of nitrogen containing dietary intake that leads to an equal nitrogen excretion – a steady-state mass balance. Although used for years, and the basis for the current Dietary Reference Intakes report[372] and FAO report[373] on protein and amino acid intake recommendations such as the RDA, this method has

---

[372] Dietary Reference Intakes (2005) Institute of Medicine, Food and Nutrition Board, Dietary Reference Intakes: Energy, Carbohydrate, Fiber, fat, Fatty Acids, Cholesterol, Protein and Amino Acids. Washington, DC: The National Academy Press.

[373] Food and Agricultural Organization (2007) Protein and amino acid requirements in human nutrition. Report of a joint WHO/FAO/UNU expert consultation. WHO Technical Report Series, No. 935. Geneva, Switzerland.

been criticized[374] including a general predisposition to overestimate nitrogen intake and underestimate nitrogen excretion, which together could result in an underestimation of true protein requirements[375].

A newer technique for estimation of protein requirements, the indicator amino acid oxidation method, is thought to be more accurate and suggests advantages of a higher protein intake as well as substantially higher EAA intake[376].

According to the above referenced Institute of Medicine, Food and Nutrition Board and the WHO's Food and Agricultural Organization, the Recommended Daily Allowance (RDA) for protein should be in the vicinity of 0.8 g/kg body weight or more. For example, a person weighing 155 pounds (70 kg) is recommended to consume on the average about 56 grams per day of protein. The protein needs of the very young (less than one year old) and older adults (over 60 years) may be somewhat greater than the population with ages in-between, and are recommended to be about 1.5 g/kg and 1.0 g/kg, respectively.

However, other research suggests that the requirement for total dietary protein is not different for healthy older adults than for younger adults and that the allowance estimate does

---

[374] Millward, D. J. (2001). Methodological considerations. *Proceedings of the Nutrition Society Proc. Nutr. Soc., 60*(01), 3-5. doi:10.1079/pns200064.

[375] Bistrian, B. (n.d.). Faculty of 1000 evaluation for Reevaluation of the protein requirement in young men with the indicator amino acid oxidation technique.*F1000 - Post-publication Peer Review of the Biomedical Literature*. doi:10.3410/f.1093982.548933.

[376] Elango, R., Ball, R. O., & Pencharz, P. B. (2012). Recent advances in determining protein and amino acid requirements in humans. *British Journal of Nutrition Br J Nutr, 108*(S2). doi:10.1017/s0007114512002504.

not differ statistically from the RDA[377]. The complexities of how much consumed protein is actually bioavailable and the variances of individual metabolism and needs, all combine to make general statements on protein requirements difficult.

HOW MUCH PROTEIN AND ESSENTIAL AMINO ACIDS ARE TYPICAL IN AMERICAN DIETS?

All EAAs originate from plants. All plants have all EAAs. Those living on a plant-based diet average about twice the RDA for protein.

You have undoubtedly heard that unless one eats animals and/ or animal products, one will have insufficient intake of protein. There appears to be a protein marketing hysteria. But it is very unlikely that, whatever your dietary pattern, you are below the RDA for protein.

Consider, for example, the cross-sectional study of the nutrient profiles of vegetarian and non-vegetarian dietary patterns of over 70,000 participants that revealed non-vegetarians (meat eaters) had the lowest intakes of plant proteins, fiber, beta carotene, and magnesium compared to those following vegetarian dietary patterns, and the highest intakes of saturated, trans, arachidonic, and other unhealthy fatty acids[378].

That's no surprise but what was quite notable was that the total protein intake among non vegetarians (meat eaters),

---

[377] *W W Campbell, C A Johnson, G P McCabe, N S Carnell. Dietary protein requirements of younger and older adults. Am J Clin Nutr. 2008 Nov;88(5):1322-9.*

[378] Rizzo, N. S., Jaceldo-Siegl, K., Sabate, J., & Fraser, G. E. (2013). Nutrient Profiles of Vegetarian and Nonvegetarian Dietary Patterns. *Journal of the Academy of Nutrition and Dietetics, 113*(12), 1610-1619. doi:10.1016/ j.jand.2013.06.349.

"semi-vegetarians", pesco vegetarian, lacto-ovo vegetarians, and strict vegetarians was quite similar at about 70 grams per day. That's well over the RDA.

COULD YOU BE PROTEIN DEFICIENT?

Not unless you are in an advanced stage of starvation. The symptoms are most commonly seen in nutritionaly deprived children in poor countries. Where protein intake is exceptionally low, there are physical signs - stunting, poor musculature, edema, thin and fragile hair, and skin lesions. Edema and loss of muscle mass and hair are the most prominent signs in adults. Deficiency of this severity is *very rare* in the United States, except as a consequence of pathologic conditions and poor medical management of the acutely ill.

> *While total protein requirements are disputed, it is unlikely your total protein intake will ever be insufficient regardless of your dietary mix.*

Even under the extreme condition of a protein-free diet, protein synthesis and breakdown continue by reutilizing amino acids. However, there is a so-called *obligatory* nitrogen loss through excretion and so amino acid stores are slowly catabolized so eventually, after months of a no-protein diet, there could develop signs of deficiency.

THE OPTIMAL PROTEIN DIET

We may be getting ample protein to satisfy the RDA, but what is the *optimal* protein intake?

It is known that our livers can store the various essential amino acids so it's not critical to combine different protein sources at each meal, perhaps not even over the course of a single day or several days. The 2009 American Dietetic Association's Position Paper on Vegetarian Diets, states[379]:

> *"Plant protein can meet requirements when a variety of plant foods is consumed and energy needs are met. Research indicates that an assortment of plant foods eaten over the course of a day can provide all EAAs and ensure adequate retention and use in healthy adults, thus complementary proteins do not need to be consumed at the same meal."*

The most important thing to be aware of regarding protein in diets devoid of any animals or animal products, the whole-food varied-plant diet, is not the total daily protein, in fact not the EAA mix, but the essential amino acid *lysine*. If you are getting the RDA for lysine, almost certainly you are getting enough protein and all other EAAs. Per serving, legumes and seitan are the foods highest in lysine.

DO YOU KNOW BEANS?

The table below contains the RDA for EAAs. Also shown is an example of the total RDA for a person weighing 155 pounds (70 kg); next to that are the EAAs from one can (16 oz) of black beans.

---

[379] Position of the American Dietetic Association: Vegetarian Diets. (2009). *Journal of the American Dietetic Association, 109*(7), 1266-1282. doi:10.1016/j.jada.2009.05.027.

Figure 7 Essential Amino Acids Daily Requirements

essential amino acid	mg/kg day required	for 155 lb person, mg/day	one can black beans, mg
histidine	11	1705	2558
isoleucine	15	2325	3488
leucine	34	5270	7905
lysine	31	4805	7208
methionine	15	2325	3488
phenylalanine	27	4185	6278
threonine	16	2480	3720
tryptophan	4	620	930
valine	19	2945	4418

As can be seen, one can of black beans easily provides all of the RDA EAAs. Generally, most beans, and more generally legumes, provide high protein and EAA content. A meal that contains legumes or beans each day is a very good way to assure excellent whole-food protein intake with all EAAs.

If your total caloric intake is low on a particular day but your protein intake is good, your cells can convert excess protein to molecules that can burn as fuel. On the other hand, if you consume plenty of calories including excess protein, your body has no choice but to convert the extra protein to fatty acids and store them in your adipose tissue.

In whole-food varied-plant diets, variety is the key to healthy eating – hence the inclusion of "varied-plant" into the name for this dietary pattern. To get all the essential nutrients, it is important to eat fruits, vegetables, nuts, seeds, legumes, whole-grain cereals, and soy products. It is important to choose plant foods that are carefully grown and stored to maintain their nutrient content.

PROTEIN QUALITY

The term "protein quality" refers to having the essential amino acids in the proper proportions. If one or more amino acids are not present in sufficient amounts, the protein in a food is considered "incomplete." This is a misleading concept. First of all, there is no established benefit in having a certain percentage amino acid mix in a given food, only that there are some amounts of each essential amino acid present, and there always are. So if a given food has a relatively low amount of a certain EAA, an increase in the total quantity of that food may remedy that issue.

Not only does a given meal not need to have a "balanced" EAA mix, or even a total RDA for an EAA, as a later meal that day or perhaps even the next day can be sufficient to cover the EAA RDA. Or a previous collection of EAA can be utilized because amino acids are stored in the liver for a time. There is an effective "pool" of EAAs ready to deliver[380].

There is yet another "buffering" system that allows poor EAA intake over a sustained length of time. It's called *gut luminal endogenous protein*[381]. Endogenous protein is non-dietary protein from our bodily sources of saliva, gastric secretions, bile, sloughed epithelia cells, plasma proteins – even significant protein from gut microbes. There may average as much as 90 grams of endogenous protein per day from which amino acids are recycled[382].

---

[380] H N Munro. CHAPTER 34 – Free Amino Acid Pools and Their Role in Regulation. Mammalian Protein Metabolism. 1970. 299–386.

[381] Moughan, P. J., & Rutherfurd, S. M. (2012). Gut luminal endogenous protein: Implications for the determination of ileal amino acid digestibility in humans. *British Journal of Nutrition Br J Nutr, 108*(S2). doi:10.1017/s0007114512002474.

[382] Ibid.

OTHER SPECIAL PROTEIN REQUIREMENTS

It has been recommended that highly active individuals such as endurance athletes should consume protein greater than the RDA of 0.8 g/kg, developed for healthy non-exercising populations. The protein intake recommendation for such individuals is 1.2 – 1.4 g/kg day based on the nitrogen balance

> *It is important to consume adequate amounts of essential amino acids for neurotransmitter synthesis in the brain.*

method[383]; newer indicator amino acid oxidation methods recommend daily protein intake as high as 1.8 g/kg[384] for those highly active.

The so-called "window of anabolic opportunity" refers to the time interval following moderate to heavy physical conditioning in which certain muscle groups are beginning a reconstruction after breakdown from strenuous exercise. Generally, the sooner new protein (and other nutrients including carbohydrates and water) can begin to be brought to task the better but likely the window is open for at least 24-hours[385]. Also rather than a sudden bolus of high protein intake, a more

---

[383] Position of the American Dietetic Association, Dietitians of Canada, and the American College of Sports Medicine: Nutrition and Athletic Performance. (2009). *Journal of the American Dietetic Association, 109*(3), 509-527. doi:10.1016/j.jada.2009.01.005.

[384] Kato, H., Suzuki, K., Bannai, M., & Moore, D. R. (2016). Protein Requirements Are Elevated in Endurance Athletes after Exercise as Determined by the Indicator Amino Acid Oxidation Method. *PLOS ONE PLoS ONE, 11*(6). doi:10.1371/journal.pone.0157406.

[385] Burd, N. A., Tang, J. E., Moore, D. R., & Phillips, S. M. (2008). Exercise training and protein metabolism: Influences of contraction, protein intake, and sex-based differences. *Journal of Applied Physiology, 106*(5), 1692-1701. doi:10.1152/japplphysiol.91351.2008.

gradual, extended intake is more likely to be assimilated. See Chapter 13 for suggestions on how to do that.

There is little evidence that mild muscular activity, such as walking, increases the need for protein, except for the small amount required for mild to moderate physical conditioning[386]. In view of the margin of safety in the RDA, no additional incremental protein intake is necessary.

No added allowance is necessary for the usual stresses encountered in daily living, which can give rise to transient increases in urinary nitrogen output. It is assumed that the subjects of experiments forming the basis for the RDA estimates are usually exposed to the same stresses as the population generally.

Extreme environmental or physiological stress such as from infections, fevers, accidents, and surgical trauma increases nitrogen loss and increases the need for protein, dependent on the degree of physiologic stress.

LIFE, DEATH, AND PROTEINS

Eating relatively little protein and lots of carbohydrates, the opposite of what's urged by many diet plans, including the popular Atkins Diet, extends life and fortifies health, including assisting mental health.

Calorie restriction, a diet that helps humans and other species live much longer than normal, may work not because it slashes caloric intake, but mostly because it cuts down on protein. This

---

[386] Torun, B., N.S. Scrimshaw, and V.R. Young. 1977. Effect of isometric exercises on body potassium and dietary protein requirements of young men. Am. J. Clin. Nutr. 30: 1983–1993.

was illustrated in a large study of the effect of low-protein intake which showed a significant decrease in mortality[387]:

> *"Respondents ... reporting high protein intake had a 75% increase in overall mortality and a 4-fold increase in cancer and diabetes mortality during an 18 year follow up period. These associations were either abolished or attenuated if the source of proteins was plant-based ... "*

Among subjects with no diabetes at baseline, those in the high protein group had a 73-fold increase in risk; while those in the moderate protein category had an almost 23-fold increase in the risk of diabetes mortality:

> *"Our results show strong significant associations between increased protein intake and diabetes-related mortality."*

These comparisons of "high" and "moderate" protein intake to "low" protein intake therefore results in my recommendation of the lower protein intake of 15% of calories from protein.

---

[387] Levine, M., Suarez, J., Brandhorst, S., Balasubramanian, P., Cheng, C., Madia, F., . . . Longo, V. (2014). Low Protein Intake Is Associated with a Major Reduction in IGF-1, Cancer, and Overall Mortality in the 65 and Younger but Not Older Population. *Cell Metabolism, 19*(3), 407-417. doi:10.1016/j.cmet.2014.02.006.

CHAPTER 11

Carbohydrates

"Only the wisest and stupidest of men never change."

Confucius

OUR CRITICAL ENERGY SOURCE

We have previously explored some aspects of two macronutrients, fat and protein. In the context of animals and animal products as food, those two macronutrients can rather much be separated as individual entities. For example, an ounce of bacon fat is 100% fat – no protein, no carbohydrates, no vitamins or minerals. Very lean animal muscle tissue consists primarily of protein and fat (75% protein and 25% fat in the leanest of portions) but no carbohydrates, essentially no vitamins, only a modicum of minerals, and a lot of harmful constituents such as cholesterol, arachidonic acids, endotoxins, etc., that we have previously detailed.

But when we consider plant foods, there is *always* a blend of all the macronutrients plus vitamins, minerals, and phytonutrients. It can be somewhat misleading to take one nutrient out of this context, such as carbohydrates (reductionist thinking) rather than considering the whole.

Nevertheless, with this in mind, we shall discuss the third macronutrient and most important energy source, carbohydrates.

Carbohydrates consist of three general types: sugars, starches, and fiber. Sugars are the simple basic building blocks for the more complex carbohydrates, much as fatty acids for fats and amino acids for protein.

The two main sugars are glucose and fructose. All plants make glucose during photosynthesis; plants store glucose by joining these simple sugars into long chains called starch. Glucose circulates in the human bloodstream as blood sugar and a certain amount can be stored in the liver for ready access in the form of glycogen.

> *Glucose is essentially the sole energy source for brain metabolism.*

Glucose is essentially the sole energy source[388] for brain metabolism and the brain generally has priority over other organs and tissue for its utilization.

---

[388] Under certain conditions – such as starvation - the brain can use "ketone bodies" in place of glucose as substrates. Ketone bodies are formed from catabolism of fatty acids by the liver.

MENTAL EFFORT

Mental effort has been described as energy mobilization in the service of cognitive goals[389]. The increase of mental effort represents a compensatory strategy to sustain performance in the presence of increased task demands and psychological stressors.

Complex carbohydrates in the context of plant foods supply glucose in a slowly released manner.

One might think of two categories of mental effort investment: "immediate effort" being a response to high surges of demands (such as time pressure, multi-tasking, high working memory load), and "sustained effort" required to protect performance from the potential negative influences of mental fatigue, sleep deprivation, and noise, as some examples.

Because our brains have a substantial glucose energy requirement under normal conditions (20 – 30% of the total energy requirements for an individual at rest) and we cannot store glucose, we need a constant supply. Additional substantial mental effort requires additional glucose. Experiments have correlated the degree of glucose responsiveness with the effectiveness of mental effort[390].

---

[389] Gaillard, A.W.K., 2001. Stress, workload, and fatigue as three biobehavioural states: a general overview. In: Hancock, P.A., Desmond, P.A. (Eds.), Stress, Workload, and Fatigue. Erlbaum, Mahweh, NJ, pp. 623–639.

[390] Fairclough, Stephen H.; Houston, Kim (2004), "A metabolic measure of mental effort", *Biol. Psychol.*, 66 *(2)*: 177–90.

Changes in mood have also been linked to fluctuating levels of blood glucose[391]; for instance, there is increased tension with a decline of blood glucose[392]. These findings suggest that the affective costs of effort may result from declining blood glucose.

DESPERATELY SEEKING FIBER

While plants have no skeletal system per se, they do have a rigid enough structure to keep them upright. This is primarily a result of their rigid cell walls, discussed briefly earlier as an evolutionary choice a strain of eukaryotes happened to make. Technically, it's not just the rigidity of the cell wall, but the tensile strength of the wall combined with hydraulic pressure from within the cell that keeps it rigid. Observe a plant wilting from lack of water to illustrate.

The plant cell wall performs many functions besides structure and thus its chemical composition is somewhat complex; certainly the major constituent of the cell wall of green plants is cellulose, the most abundant organic polymer on earth.

It used to be, as we learned in high school, cellulose was equated to fiber, and fiber in the diet was primarily a consideration for regularity in bowel movement. But there is much more to the story than that.

Even the definition of *fiber* is not consistently accepted[393]. First fiber was defined as the components of plants that resist

---

[391] Benton, D. (2002). Carbohydrate ingestion, blood glucose and mood. *Neuroscience & Biobehavioral Reviews, 26*(3), 293-308. doi:10.1016/ s0149-7634(02)00004-0.

[392] Ibid.

[393] Consider those of the Institute of Medicine (Institute of Medicine; Food and Nutrition Board. Dietary Reference Intakes: energy, carbohydrates, fiber, fat, fatty acids, cholesterol, protein and amino acids. Wash-

human digestive enzymes, a definition that added to cellulose other material such as lignin, a "woody" organic polymer not quite as plentiful as cellulose. The next addition to the definition of fiber were certain water-soluble materials that were easily fermented by gut bacteria and resulted in physiologically active prebiotic by-products. Then a third class considered by some as a fiber was "resistant starch", those starches that resist digestion and absorption in the small intestine.

It would seem now that fiber is defined basically as plant material that can influence the functioning of the gastrointestinal tract, including the microbiome by changing how other nutrients are absorbed. So fiber is far from being inert substances that go along for the ride so you can go along to the bathroom.

While human enzymes may not be able to digest dietary fiber, it is digestible by our gut bacteria, which make short-chain fatty acids from it, inhibiting the growth of harmful gut bacteria, increasing mineral absorption such as calcium, stimulating blood flow as well as colonic fluid and electrolyte uptake. Furthermore, there may be digestible phytonutrients that are chemically attached to the fibrous content and released during

> *Dietary fiber helps maintain a favorable microbiome and is important in proper cholesterol balance and elimination.*

---

ington (DC): National Academies Press; 2005.) and that of the Codex Alimentarius Commission (Codex Alimentarius Commission; Food and Agriculture Organization; World Health Organization. Report of the 30th session of the Codex Committee on nutrition and foods for special dietary uses. ALINORM 9/32/26. 2009).

processing by our micro flora[394].

There may be an additional evolutionary effect from millions of years of primates consuming significant amounts of fiber: *satiation*. Diets high in fiber do fill the stomach and reduce the drive to eat. A diet low in fiber but energy dense would lead to extra caloric consumption prior to satiation. If this becomes a consistent pattern, as in diets currently in Western cultures, it contributes to obesity.

Soluble fiber forms a kind of a gel in water that helps bind acids and cholesterol in the intestinal tract, preventing their re-absorption into the body. This may be why soluble fiber helps to lower cholesterol levels. Excess cholesterol is dumped into the bowel, adheres to fiber and exits. Without sufficient fiber, and the great majority of Westerners are very deficient in fiber, that excess cholesterol is reabsorbed. Soluble fiber is found in oats and oat bran, barley, brown rice, beans, apples, carrots, and most other fruits and vegetables.

> *We evolved to experience meal satiation in part because of significant fiber consumption, now deficient in modern dietary patterns.*

---

[394] Arranz, S., Silván, J., & Saura-Calixto, F. (2010). Nonextractable polyphenols, usually ignored, are the major part of dietary polyphenols: A study on the Spanish diet. *Molecular Nutrition & Food Research Mol. Nutr. Food Res.*, 54(11), 1646-1658.

CHAPTER 12

Macronutrient Distribution

"Don't dig your grave with your own knife and fork".

English Proverb

CALORIC MACRONUTRIENT DISTRIBUTION

Based on our recommendations for total fat (Chapter 9) and protein (Chapter 10), a reasonable recommended caloric intake for these macronutrients is 10% and 15% per day, respectively. That results, by summation of 10% plus 15% and subtraction from 100%, in one's daily caloric intake to be 75% from carbohydrates, illustrated in the chart below and agreeing with that suggested in our earlier book The New Ancestral Diet, based on evolution. Of course, the thinking behind these overall percentages must be kept in mind: the need for correct distributions of essential fats, adequate essential amino acids, and complex nutritive carbohydrates with fiber.

Figure 8 The New Ancestral Diet Macronutrient Distribution

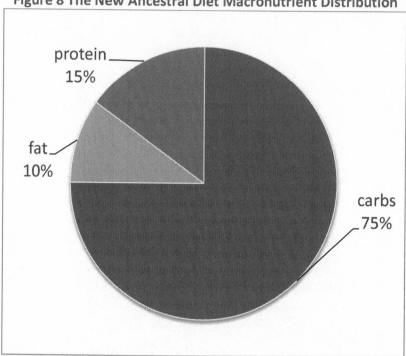

This distribution is consistent with that suggested, for example, by Neal Barnard, of the Physicians Committee for Responsible Medicine, for a whole-food plant-based diet that primates have subsisted on throughout their evolution, including the great majority of the Paleolithic Period.

While some may argue that 15% protein is too low, consider the fact that human breast milk, a whole-food complete diet composition designed by nature as most nourishing, contains only 8% protein. Of course, the needs of infants difer from those of older individuals, but this is the only absolute indication of optimal nutritional requirements of a human, so is mentioned here.

This is quite different from the Standard American Diet (SAD) shown below, the difference being in the relatively high fat content, including large amounts of "bad" fats. The carbohydrate mix includes a large percentage of simple added sugars.

Figure 9 SAD Macronutrient Composition

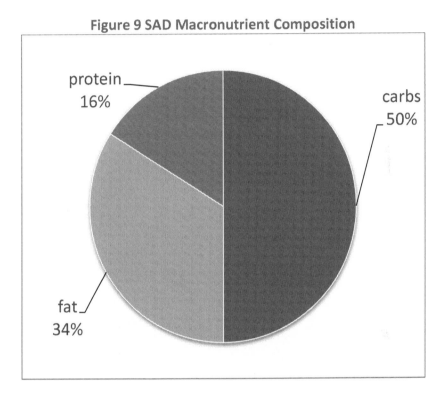

THE OKINAWA TRADITIONAL DIET

People of the Okinawa archipelago in Japan consume the traditional diet of that region – they also have one of the highest longevity rates in the world.

In addition to their long life expectancy, these islanders are noted for their low mortality from vascular disease (eight times less than Americans) and certain types of cancers, such as prostate, breast, and colon cancers.

Other factors in addition to diet undoubtedly contribute to the longevity of Okinawan centenarians. Most grew a garden and participated in daily physical activity. Tending a garden also lowers stress and increases vitamin D intake.

Their macronutrient mix is shown in the following chart:

Figure 10 The Okinawa Diet Macronutrient Distribution

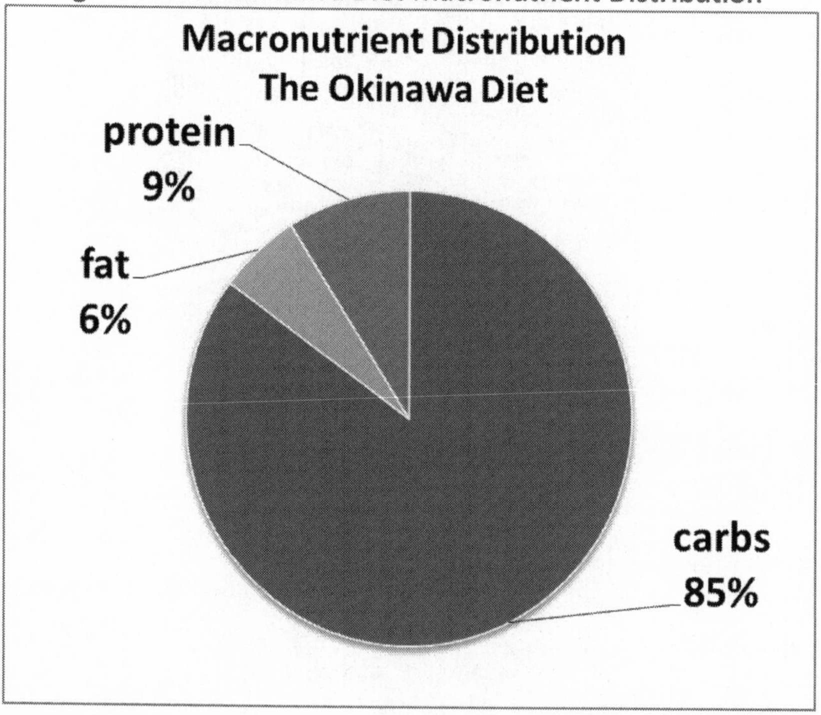

This indicates an even lower percentage of fat in total caloric intake, but otherwise similar to our recommendations.

The three illustrated dietary patterns are shown below using a *right angle mixture* (RAM) triangle graphic:

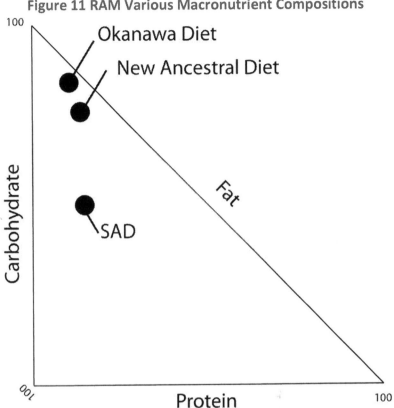

Figure 11 RAM Various Macronutrient Compositions

It can be seen that the relative macronutrient composition mix for our recommended diet is close to that of the Okinawa diet but much different from the SAD.

ENERGY DENSITY VERSUS NUTRIENT DENSITY

The main activity of our ancestral primates has been eating – acquiring calories for energy. Energy-dense foods, therefore, have been favored to assure adequate caloric intake.

This is no longer an issue in Western society from a food availability standpoint. Nevertheless, energy-density is still favored in the SAD over *nutrient density*.

Consider the following graph on which energy density and nutrient density are indicated for a number of different foods. "Percent max" on the ordinate is based on pure fat as 100% energy dense; percent max for nutrient density is based on the measure used by Nutrition Data[395].

Figure 12 Energy Density and Nutrient Density

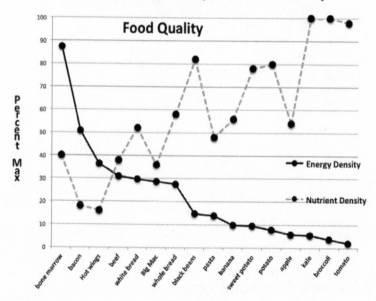

Generally there is an inverse relationship between energy density and nutrient density.

---

[395] There are many ways to measure nutrient density and no universally acceptable way. This measure used here does not include the phytonutrients so is a lower limit on nutrition. (n.d.). Retrieved May 28, 2015, from http://nutritiondata.self.com.

Those foods favored by the SAD include those of highest energy density such as bacon, hot wings, beef, and the Big Mac. Those of the highest nutrient density include tomatoes, broccoli, and kale.

A choice of foods based on cut-off points for these two parameters might be: energy density less than 20% and nutrient density greater than 40%. That effectively eliminates animal products and refined grains.

The graph below illustrates the ratio of nutrient density (as defined above) to energy density for select fruits and vegetables.

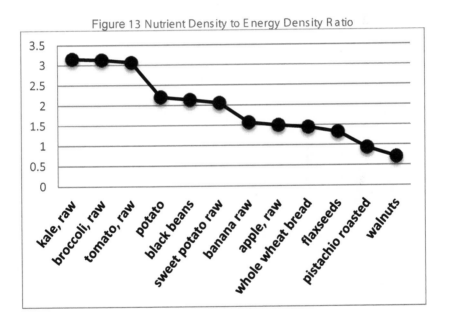

Figure 13 Nutrient Density to Energy Density Ratio

There can be seen on the plot a couple of plateaus – the first, at the highest ratio, contains typical green vegetables; the second legumes and underground storage organs; the next fruits; and finally grains, seeds and nuts. Basically, this is the order of priority *in quantity* we recommend when constructing a daily menu.

A NOTE ON THE DEFINITION OF NUTRIENT DENSITY

There is no accepted definition of nutrient density. Most definitions involve merely selecting nutrients, sometimes including protein as a macronutrient, and certain vitamins and minerals, then dividing by an RDA for each of those nutrients. The sum of each selected nutrient for a given food, possibly divided by its caloric value, is then related to the nutrient density of that food. This presupposes that the RDA is meaningful. It does not address the phytonutrient content, for example, anti-oxidants, anti-inflammatories, alkalinity, fiber, or glycemic index.

Most importantly, this reductionist approach that breaks down individual nutrients out of the context of the whole can be misleading. For example, a multivitamin pill could score extremely high in nutrient density although it has never been shown to be effective unless an individual has a (rare) nutrient deficiency and even then would not be the treatment of choice.

Part IV WHERE

Where do you find specific foods for health and happiness of mind and body?

CHAPTER 13

Good Mood Food

"An undefined problem has an indefinite number of solutions."

Robert A. Humphrey

WHOLE-FOOD VARIED-PLANTS

The dietary pattern suggested in this book is whole-food varied-plants. Because of an emphasis on mental wellness in addition to physical health, there are certain dietary elements that are particularly encouraged.

We shall go through each of the pathological conditions contributing to cognitive decline and emotional illness and indicate for each condition specifically what dietary interventions you can make.

CEREBROVASCULAR DISEASE AND CHOLESTEROL

As mentioned in Chapter 4, the central single causative factor in the creation of vascular disease, including cardiovascular and cerebrovascular disease as well as vascular disease of all other organs, is cholesterol. Cholesterol is produced by all animal cells because it is an essential component to the structural integrity of the cell membrane; this allows animal cells to change shape and animals to move. Plants, on the other hand, do not manufacture cholesterol so substitution of a diet rich in plants rather than animal products effectively lowers cholesterol.

While cholesterol is a vital compound that our body produces, it does so in a balanced feed-back controlled way. Taking on the cholesterol of other animals contributes significantly to the leading causes of death and morbidity in the Western world. There is also an inflammatory process that utilizes cholesterol resulting in occlusion or buildup and break-off of diseased tissue but we shall reflect on inflammation in a later section of this chapter.

Obviously, the dietary pattern that directly contributes to increased cholesterol, eating of animal flesh, is to be eliminated. Even the National Science Academies states[396]:

> *"All (of our) tissues are capable of synthesizing enough cholesterol to meet their metabolic and structural needs. Consequently, there is no evidence for a biological requirement for dietary cholesterol. ... Much evidence indicates a positive linear trend between cholesterol*

---

[396] Food and Nutrition Board. (2005). *Dietary reference intakes for energy, carbohydrate, fiber, fat, fatty acids, cholesterol, protein, and amino acids* (p. 423). Washington, D.C.: National Academies Press.

intake and low density lipoprotein (LDL) cholesterol concentration, and therefore an increased risk of coronary heart disease (and all vascular disease such as cerebrovascular disease). *A Tolerable Upper Intake Level (UL) was not set for cholesterol because any incremental increase in cholesterol intake increases risk. It is recommended that people maintain their dietary cholesterol intake as low as possible."*

"As low as possible" is zero.

Recall that gradual deterioration in the tissue served by the very high degree of vascularization in the brain, neurons being much more sensitive to oxygen deprivation than other types of cells, can lead to damage to the brain with life changing effects on our cognition, emotions, and behavior.

DIETARY INTERVENTIONS FOR CEREBROVASCULAR DISEASE

Obviously a whole-food varied-plant diet is indicated to reduce vascular disease. But are there specific dietary components that might alone or in combination be particularly helpful?

There is substantial evidence from randomized controlled trials that a number of foods can significantly reduce LDL-cholesterol. These foods have traditionally been considered as a single addition to a lipid-modification diet.

Garlic

Hippocrates prescribed garlic for a variety of medical conditions. Garlic was given to the original Olympic athletes in

Greece as perhaps one of the earliest "performance enhancing" agents[397].

In India, three ancient medical traditions, i.e., Tibbi, Unani and Ayurvedic, made extensive use of garlic as a central part of the healing efficacy of plants. The leading surviving medical text, *Charaka-Samhita*, recommended garlic for the treatment of vascular disease and arthritis 2000 years ago.

A leading physician during the latter part of the 12th century, the Abbess of Rupertsberg, St. Hildegard von Bingen, focused on garlic in her medical writing. She came to the conclusion that raw garlic had more health benefits than cooked garlic, a point of view verified more recently.

Garlic, and to a much lesser extent other allium vegetables such as onions and chives, has been found to lower cholesterol, prevent blood clots, reduce blood pressure, and protect against infections[398]. Now research has found that it helps stop artery-clogging plaque at its earliest stage. Garlic keeps individual cholesterol particles from sticking to artery walls.

Garlic helps to lower cholesterol. Use liberally.

These advantages are for raw garlic and onions – cooking reduces the benefits[399].

---

[397] Green, O., & Polydoris, N. (1993). *Garlic, cancer and heart disease: Review and recommendations* (pp. 21-41). Chicago, Ill.: GN Communications (Pub.).

[398] Lau, K. -., Chan, Y. -., Wong, Y. -., Teo, K. -., Yiu, K. -., Liu, S., . . . Tse, H. F. (2013). Garlic intake is an independent predictor of endothelial function in patients with ischemic stroke. *J Nutr Health Aging The Journal of Nutrition, Health & Aging, 17*(7), 600-604. doi:10.1007/s12603-013-0043-6.

[399] Ali, M., Bordia, T., & Mustafa, T. (1999). Effect of raw versus boiled aqueous extract of garlic and onion on platelet aggrega-

As most garlic and onions are cooked at high temperatures as a flavoring for many dishes, there are two biohacks that can preserve much of the health benefits. The first is to crush or mince the garlic and wait ten minutes or more because the enzyme that catalyzes the anti-platelet activity is activated by the crushing but deactivated by cooking[400]. The other is to add a little raw garlic to microwaved-uncrushed garlic with subsequent crushing[401].

Plant sterols and stanols

There is extensive literature that has evaluated the effects of plant stanols and sterols on blood lipids. Plant sterols and stanols are naturally occurring compounds structurally similar to cholesterol with a cellular function similar to human cholesterol. Research estimates that 1.5–1.9 grams of plant sterols per day and 2.0–2.4 grams of plant stanols per day is enough to reduce LDL-cholesterol by an average of 8.5 and 8.9 %, respectively. This has FDA approval in the United States[402] and a granted health claim in Europe by the European Safety Authority[403].

---

tion. *Prostaglandins, Leukotrienes and Essential Fatty Acids (PLEFA), 60*(1), 43-47. doi:10.1054/plef.1998.0006.

[400] Cavagnaro, P. F., & Galmarini, C. R. (2012). Effect of Processing and Cooking Conditions on Onion (Allium cepa L.) Induced Antiplatelet Activity and Thiosulfinate Content. *J. Agric. Food Chem. Journal of Agricultural and Food Chemistry, 60*(35), 8731-8737. doi:10.1021/jf301793b.

[401] Cavagnaro, P. F., Camargo, A., Galmarini, C. R., & Simon, P. W. (2007). Effect of Cooking on Garlic (Allium sativum L.) Antiplatelet Activity and Thiosulfinates Content. *J. Agric. Food Chem. Journal of Agricultural and Food Chemistry, 55*(4), 1280-1288. doi:10.1021/jf062587s.

[402] Food and Drug Administration (2000) Food labeling: health claims; plant sterol/stanol esters and coronary heart disease; interim final rule http://www.fda.gov/Food/ LabelingNutrition/ LabelClaims/ Health-ClaimsMeetingSignificantScientificAgreementSSA/ucm074747.htm.

[403] European Food Safety Authority (2009) Scientific opinion: Plant stanols and plant sterols and blood LDL-cholesterol. Scientific opinion of

Supplements are available that contain both plant sterols and stanols and cost about $0.30 for a daily dose of 3.6 grams. This is against the "whole-food" ethic; also in the above referenced research trials, sterols and stanols were in the form of "enriched" plant fat dairy spreads, mayonnaise, salad dressing, milk and yoghurt[404], but is also available in pure supplement form. The concentrations necessary for the therapeutic effect just cannot be obtained from whole foods. When it comes to reducing the number one cause of death in the Western world, exceptions to the whole – food ethic might be considered.

Soy protein

The literature relating to soy protein lowering LDL-cholesterol is extensive, with over one-hundred randomized controlled trials and a large number of meta-analyses. Analysis of the meta-analyses would indicate that regular intake of 25 grams of soy protein per day reduces LDL-cholesterol about 5.5%.

An analysis of 47 studies evaluated the effects of food from soy protein on LDL-cholesterol lowering. It was concluded that different food forms of soy protein did not have significantly differing effects on net reductions of LDL-cholesterol when isolated soy protein was compared with soy protein from soy milk, tofu, or other food forms. However, a typical cup of

---

the Panel on Dietetic Products, Nutrition and Allergies on a request from the European Commission and a similar request from France in relation to the authorization procedure for health claims on plant stanols and plant sterols and lowering/reducing blood LDL-cholesterol pursuant to Article 14 of Regulation (EC) no 1924/ 2006. Opinion of the Panel on Dietetic Products, Nutrition and Allergies. EFSA J 1175, 1–9.

[404] Abumweis, S. S., Barake, R., & Jones, P. (2008). Plant sterols/stanols as cholesterol lowering agents: A meta-analysis of randomized controlled trials.*Food & Nutrition Research, 52*(0). doi:10.3402/fnr.v52i0.1811.

soymilk has only about 8 grams of protein, so to meet the 25 mg daily requirement would require three cups.

Soy protein, a "complete" protein, is available as a powder; 25 mg is about one third of a cup of powder (more than five tablespoons) and costs about $0.60 per serving (100 calories). That's too much to cram into capsules.

Soluble fiber

Sources of soluble fiber from oats and barley have shown definite cholesterol lowering properties, mainly from ß-glucans. Oat ß-glucans behave as a prebiotic: a non-digestible food ingredient that beneficially affects the host by selectively stimulating the growth and/or activity of one strain or a limited number of bacterial strains in the colon and thus improving host health[405]. ß-glucans decompose in the large intestine.

For a significant LDL cholesterol lowering effect, foods containing at least 3 grams of ß-glucans per day, such as from oats, oat bran, barley, or barley bran can lower LDL cholesterol by 7% or more. To achieve this level of ß-glucan intake, cereals required is about 84 g/day corresponding roughly to a full cup of oats, oat bran, barley, or barley bran.

Tree nuts

Epidemiologic studies have consistently demonstrated an association between tree nut consumption and coronary heart disease (CHD) morbidity and mortality in different

---

[405] Daou, C., & Zhang, H. (2012). Oat Beta-Glucan: Its Role in Health Promotion and Prevention of Diseases. *Comprehensive Reviews in Food Science and Food Safety, 11*(4), 355-365. doi:10.1111/j.1541-4337.2012.00189.x.

populations[406]. Compared to people who ate nuts less than once per week, those who ate them one to four times per week had a 25% reduced risk of dying from CHD; people who ate nuts more than five 5 times per week experienced about a 50% reduction in risk[407]. These benefits are officially acknowledged by the United States Federal Drug Administration[408].

Nuts are a good source of unsaturated fatty acids, both monounsaturated fatty acids (MUFA) and PUFA, known for their favorable effects on blood lipids. Furthermore, evidence suggests that components in nuts further reduce LDL cholesterol concentrations beyond the effects based solely on fatty acid profiles[409]. Therefore, the possible mechanisms whereby nuts may improve lipid profiles may include a multitude of whole nut effects of fiber (about 25% soluble), micronutrients such as vitamin E and C, folic acid, copper, magnesium, selenium, plant protein (e.g., arginine), plant sterols, and phenolic components.

Consumption of 50–100 g/ day of nuts, especially almonds, Brazil, peanuts, pecans, or walnuts (not so much macadamia nuts), significantly lowered LDL-cholesterol (2–19%) to a

---

[406] Kris-Etherton, P. M., Zhao, G., Binkoski, A. E., Coval, S. M. & Etherton, T. D. (2001) The effects of nuts on coronary heart disease risk. *Nutr. Rev.* 59:103-111.

[407] Dreher, M. L., Maher, C. V. & Kearney, P. (1996) The traditional and emerging role of nuts in healthful diets. *Nutr. Rev.* **54**:241-245.

[408] Brown, D. (2003) FDA considers health claim for nuts. *J. Am. Diet. Assoc.*103:426.

[409] Mensink, R. P. & Katan, M. B. (1992) Effect of dietary fatty acids on serum lipids and lipoproteins. A meta-analysis of 27 trials. *Arterioscler. Thromb.*12:911-919.

greater degree than observed for consumption of lower-fat, cholesterol-lowering diets without nuts[410].

"Portfolio" diet

A more sophisticated approach is to combine foods with enhanced cholesterol-lowering properties, the so-called "portfolio diet[411]." This terminology refers to a low-fat vegan diet enhanced by the inclusion of plant stanols or sterols, soy protein, soluble fiber and tree nuts[412].

The portfolio diet is the best way to lower your cholesterol using food.

The "portfolio" dietary components are those for which the most evidence exists for cholesterol lowering. In addition, there are a number of foods where blood lipid modification evidence is accumulating and they may have potential as cholesterol-lowering agents; these include dark chocolate, green tea, flaxseed and garlic.

It appears that the combined cholesterol lowering effect of individual components is at least additive when used in simple

---

[410] Mukuddem-Petersen, J., Oosthuizen, W., & Jerling, J. C. (2005). A Systematic Review of the Effects of Nuts on Blood Lipid Profiles in Humans. *Journal Of Nutrition*, *135*(9), 2082-2089.

[411] Jenkins, D. J., Kendall, C. W., Axelsen, M., Augustin, L. S., & Vuksan, V. (2000). Viscous and nonviscous fibres, nonabsorbable and low glycaemic index carbohydrates, blood lipids and coronary heart disease. *Current Opinion in Lipidology, 11*(1), 49-56. doi:10.1097/00041433-200002000-00008.

[412] Jenkins DJ, Kendall CW, Faulkner D, et al. (2002) A dietary portfolio approach to cholesterol reduction: combined effects of plant sterols, vegetable proteins, and viscous fibers in hypercholesterolemia. *Metabolism* 51, 1596–1604.

combinations and possibly synergistically better than the summation of each cholesterol lowering component.[413].

Typically, the portfolio dietary components contain per 1000 kcal: 1 gram of plant stanols or sterols, 16–23 grams soy protein, 8–10 grams of soluble fiber and 16 – 23 grams of tree nuts.

Where a portfolio diet is adopted the extent of the LDL cholesterol reduction is about 30 %; there does appear to be a dose-response relationship, the more one consumes each component of this diet, the better the result[414].

I have had a number of patients who follow a rather rigid no-cholesterol diet and yet cannot achieve total cholesterol under 150; some patients in this category have values well over 200. There could be a number of factors involved including genetic (as in familial hypercholesterolemia). Nevertheless, for whatever reason, if your cholesterol is above ideal and you wish to lower it beyond that which a whole-food varied-plant diet can provide, you might want to consider the portfolio diet, full or partial.

Here is one example of a quick breakfast that contains all you need for a portfolio diet meal. Prepare in the evening for a fast start in the am.

---

[413] Harland, J. I. (2012). Food combinations for cholesterol lower-ing. *Nutrition Research Reviews, 25*(02), 249-266. doi:10.1017/s0954422412000170.
[414] Ibid.

Recipe: Portfolio overnight oatmeal breakfast

- Place one cup of rolled oats into a bowl (I love my large ceramic 38 ounce bowls[415])
- Add about one cup of soy milk.
- Cover and place in refrigerator overnight (to soften the oats)
- In the morning, take out of the fridge and microwave if warmth is desired.
- Add a handful of whole or chopped almonds, Brazil, peanuts, pecans, walnuts, or a mixture of any combination of these tree nuts.
- (optional but recommended) Add some fruit, such as half a cup of blueberries.
- (optional but recommended) Mix in a tablespoon of ground flaxseeds[416] and/ or cacao nibs.

For the maximum effect, a very serious consumer who can allow the idea of a non whole-food supplement, add about one-quarter of a cup of soy powder and wash down a sterol/ stanols supplement[417] with a glass of soy milk.

EXERCISE

Although the focus in this book is on diet, when considering vascular health, exercise must be mentioned. I recommend, for those who can do it, at least 30 minutes per day of cardio

---

[415] I use Cameo Ceramic bowl, 38 Ounce, 7.25 Inch, Set of 2, White Ivory costs $25 on Amazon.

[416] One can use a coffee grinder for this; or can purchase bulk ground flaxseeds or individual packets of ground flaxseeds such as Carrington Farms organic ground milled flaxseed.

[417] For example, Nature Made CholestOff has 900 mg softgels; take two twice per day.

exercise (this should be termed "vascular" exercise but we shall use the common usage "cardio"). Use your largest muscles – those of your thighs – against gravity. The reason for use of the upper leg muscles is that other smaller muscles might fatigue before a sufficient cardio workout is achieved.

The reason I say "against gravity" is that most all cardio exercises utilize your own body weight pushing against gravity – and no extra equipment is needed. Such exercises include brisk walking, jogging, running, and climbing stairs.

Biking is another excellent cardiovascular exercise but obviously requires equipment - a bike; there are dangers in riding a bike outdoors so indoor training is safer albeit less interesting. I've had a few bike mishaps leading to rotator cuff surgeries and use an indoor trainer primarily (KICKR brand). Software such as Strava, Kinomap, Zwift, and TrainerRoad, together with the KICKR, offers visual training routes all over the world in real time with actual fellow bikers.

During my physical therapy post-shoulder surgery, I would typically "warm-up" at the rehab facility to get the circulation going in my arms and shoulder by using a machine that was much like biking with my arms, i.e. arm cranking against resistance without involving the legs, they are called simply "upper-body exercisers." I could reach over 200 watts with this device and was a cardio workout, although arm fatigue would likely limit the duration of the session for a full cardio experience. But if you have back or leg injuries, there are upper body exercises that can provide cardio; rowing is another, just concentrate on the upper body and let the back and legs go along for the ride.

Swimming is another terrific way to achieve cardio exercise. If weight bearing to the legs or other parts of the body is a limitation, the reduction of gravity through buoyancy allows movement otherwise unattainable. Swimming can be done without using the legs at all – or without using the arms at all (probably will need a kickboard for that). Just walking or jogging in the water can be excellent cardio.

I like using water resistance dumbbells (mine are Hydro-Tone Bells); the amount of "weight" is determined by the speed of movement through the water; if that is too great, just move more slowly rather than dropping the dumbbell. The range of movements is essentially infinite.

The level of effort is important. Cardio conditioning is best when the effort is at least to the level where it is somewhat difficult to carry on a normal conversation without pauses for breath.

STROKE

As detailed in Chapter 4, "stroke" refers to brain injury caused by any disruption of blood supply to the brain whether it be from vessel hemorrhage (hemorrhagic stroke) or from vessel occlusion (ischemic stroke).

Vessel occlusion is related to the vascular disease mentioned in the last section; it can originate either at the site of the brain vessel occlusion or from parts of another larger arterial occlusion that happens upstream, even in the heart itself.

Hemorrhagic stroke is most commonly related to high blood pressure. Such vessel extravasation into surrounding sensitive brain tissue (infarcts) will obviously affect the brain's function. Depending upon the degree of injury and the location, there will be varying degrees of cognitive, emotional, and behavioral decline. Multiple infarcts, even if not visible with advanced imaging technology, can lead to extreme psychiatric disorders and dementia.

BLOOD PRESSURE AND SALT

There is minimal but easily an adequate amount of salt (sodium chloride) present in a whole-food varied-plant diet. Since data were inadequate for the National Academies to calculate Recommended Daily Allowance (RDA) for sodium and chloride, Adequate Intake (AI) was given instead, 1500 mg/ day of sodium. The AI for sodium was set:

> *"at an intake that ensures that the overall diet provides an adequate intake of other important nutrients and also covers sodium sweat losses in unacclimated individuals who are exposed to high temperatures or who become physically active."*

This seems quite remarkable and inappropriate to set an adequate limit once again based on poor overall dietary patterns and special cases for an element that contributes the most to a condition that is the highest risk factor for death in the world.

High blood pressure is the highest risk factor for death in the world, and sodium is the most significant contributor.

How much sodium is in a whole-food varied-plant diet? A cup of raw kale has 29 mg of sodium; one medium size apple maybe 2 mg; a cup of black beans 10 mg; a cup of chopped broccoli 30 mg; 1 cup spouted wheat 17 mg. You get the idea. From an evolutionary standpoint, we were not meant to consume high levels of sodium; it's no surprise that doing so causes devastating health problems.

244

Be careful to limit your intake of breads and pasta, as salt is an integral ingredient in controlling the fermentation of yeast. Pizza and processed foods are loaded with salt. And please consider repurposing your salt shaker; maybe for another favorite spice.

Dredgers: all shook up

Speaking of shakers, one can purchase a number of types and sizes of dredgers: containers with small perforated holes that are used to hold herbs, spices, or other ingredients that are sprinkled on foods. Certain dredgers are made for specific spices such as cinnamon.

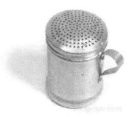

Most spices can be purchased in a small shaker container but are quite expensive. Bulk purchase of powdered cacao, garlic, cinnamon, cumin, turmeric, and many other herbs and spices each can fill a dredger, saving the remainder of the bulk in a sealed container between fillings. Even ground seeds such as flaxseeds or chia seeds could be ground in a coffee grinder, then added to a dredger. Note the oil content of ground flaxseeds once exposed to air requires use within a few weeks because of the fat content spoilage potential; best to keep in the refrigerator.

Sprinkling herbs and spices on the top surface of a food can have a pronounced effect on flavor – more than if it were mixed into the food. This is a result of the increased volatile availability in the retro-pharynx (see discussion of flavor in Chapter 8). This holds true also with spraying or drizzling juices or liquids such as Balsamic vinegars[418].

---

[418] The variety of gourmet vinegars is amazing. See online for example "The Olive Tap" that has a vast variety such as Blackberry Ginger,

NON-STEROIDAL ANTI-INFLAMMATORY DRUGS (NSAIDS)

NSAIDs, such as aspirin, ibuprofen, and naproxen, decrease synthesis of compounds called *prostaglandins*, which possess potent vasodilatory and sodium excretion effects. NSAIDs further contribute to a rise in blood pressure because they diminish the effectiveness of antihypertensive medications that involve prostaglandins, either primarily or indirectly in their mechanism of action[419].

The consumption of over-the-counter (OTC) NSAIDS is increasing, particularly as the overall mean age of the population is increasing with attendant arthritis. NSAIDs are easily and mistakenly overlooked by physicians as a source of hypertension, as they seldom appear on a reconciled medication list, being OTC. As a result, NSAIDs are most likely responsible for elevating blood pressures in many hypertensive people in the United States[420].

WEIGHT

With a whole-food varied-plant diet your weight is less likely to be an issue; if you are just starting such a dietary pattern, you undoubtedly will lose weight. Be careful to choose more nutrient-rich foods compared to energy-dense foods. Whole vegetables also have potassium that modulates the effect of

---

Pomegranate, Fig, Dark Chocolate, and their best selling Balsamic Vinegar: Aceto Balsamico di Modena, "4 Leaf Quality."

[419] Jurca, S. J., & Elliott, W. J. (2016). Common Substances That May Contribute to Resistant Hypertension, and Recommendations for Limiting Their Clinical Effects. *Current Hypertension Reports, 18*(10). doi:10.1007/s11906-016-0682-1.

[420] Elliott, W. J. (2006). Hypertension Curriculum Review Donald G. Vidt, MD, Section Editor. Drug Interactions and Drugs That Affect Blood Pressure. *The Journal of Clinical Hypertension J Clin Hypertension, 8*(10), 731-737. doi:10.1111/j.1524-6175.2006.05939.x.

sodium. A Body Mass Index[421] (BMI) less than 25 definitely helps keep blood pressure lower and should be sought.

Exercise

Exercise, as reviewed above, can help manage blood pressure. Aerobic exercise is best but strength and core work can be a great supplement to aerobics. Make it fun, as in a sport or while listening to or watching inspiring content. Once you "get into the zone" (45 minutes or more of rather intense activity), the meditative aspect of clearing the mind and just being present may be better than external recorded auditory or video content.

HABITS

Bad habits such as smoking and excessive alcohol intake significantly contribute to higher blood pressure. Good habits, once established, also are difficult to break – it works both ways.

PSYCHOLOGICAL STRESS

Chronic or dangerously acute spikes in blood pressure can result from psychological stress. Cognitive Behavioral Therapy (CBT) described in Chapter 19 can help manage that.

MONITORING

I recommend monitoring your blood pressure for safety and as a motivator if you are in the process of lowering it. Omron makes a number of excellent blood pressure self-monitors.

---

[421] BMI is a weight-to-height ratio, calculated by dividing one's weight in kilograms by the square of one's height in meters and used as an indicator of obesity and underweight.

Witherings makes a portable device activated by your smart phone and records and graphs your progress; that company also manufactures a weight scale that records, graphs, and analyzes a number of parameters including pulse wave velocity, a measure of arterial stiffness, or the rate at which pressure waves move down the arteries.

FLAXSEEDS

Four components within flaxseed may be responsible for reduction of blood pressure: ALA, lignans, fiber, peptides, or a synergistic action of all four components together. The anti-inflammatory action of ALA may explain flaxseeds' antihypertensive action[422]. Alternatively, the rich lignan content within flaxseed may provide an antihypertensive effect through its antioxidant action[423].

One prospective, double blinded, placebo controlled, randomized trial using 30 grams per day of milled flaxseed stated[424]:

> *Flaxseeds help to lower blood pressure.*

---

[422] Dupasquier, C. M., Dibrov, E., Kneesh, A. L., Cheung, P. K., Lee, K. G., Alexander, H. K., . . . Pierce, G. N. (2007). Dietary flaxseed inhibits atherosclerosis in the LDL receptor-deficient mouse in part through anti-proliferative and anti-inflammatory actions. *AJP: Heart and Circulatory Physiology, 293*(4). doi:10.1152/ajpheart.01104.2006.

[423] Prasad, K. (1997). Dietary flax seed in prevention of hypercholesterolemic atherosclerosis. *Atherosclerosis, 132*(1), 69-76. doi:10.1016/s0021-9150(97)06110-8.

[424] Rodriguez-Leyva, D., Weighell, W., Edel, A. L., Lavallee, R., Dibrov, E., Pinneker, R., . . . Pierce, G. N. (2013). Potent Antihypertensive Action of Dietary Flaxseed in Hypertensive Patients. *Hypertension, 62*(6), 1081-1089. doi:10.1161/hypertensionaha.113.02094.

"The antihypertensive effects of dietary flaxseed are potent, selective to hypertensive patients, and long-lasting. ...

and:

"In summary, flaxseed induced one of the most potent antihypertensive effects achieved by a dietary intervention."

HIBISCUS FLOWERS

Hibiscus sabdariffa L., also known as Hibiscus tea or sour tea, is a tropical wild plant rich in organic acids, polyphenols, anthocyanins, polysaccharides, and volatile constituents that are beneficial for the vascular system.

The exact mechanisms responsible for these effects of H. sabdariffa are not completely understood. Polyphenols from Hibiscus appear to induce an endothelium-dependent relaxant effect via stimulation of nitric oxide production or a decrease of blood viscosity.

> *Hibiscus flowers lower blood pressure.*

A systematic review and meta-analysis of randomized controlled trials "showed a significant effect of H. sabdariffa in lowering both systolic and diastolic blood pressure[425]." Each study averaged about 4 grams of Hibiscus in the form of aqueous extract from tea bags (each tea bag typically contains about 1.25 grams, so three tea bags); the effect was an average reduction of 7.6 mm Hg for systolic and 3.5 mm Hg for diastolic pressures. Put into perspective, the results of even a 3.3 mm Hg systolic and 1.4 mm Hg diastolic pressure reduction was

---

[425] Serban, C., Sahebkar, A., Ursoniu, S., Andrica, F., & Banach, M. (2015). Effect of sour tea (Hibiscus sabdariffa L.) on arterial hypertension. *Journal of Hypertension, 33*(6), 1119-1127. doi:10.1097/ hjh.0000000000000585.

associated with a 22% decrease of relative risk of myocardial infarction, stroke, and cardiovascular mortality[426].

Recipe: Hibiscus and green tea workout drink

Exercise and the best teas on the planet – nice combo. Adding hot water to tea bags help solubilize the polyphenols because the temperature softens the cells walls and increases the solubility of cellular contents; steeping 5 minutes or so is enough. But there is a "biohack" that can get the goodies into solution even faster: blending. The reason is that agitation in the aqueous environment and particle size reduction aids the extraction. High-speed blenders can get the particle size down below 100 microns and the agitation is maximal. Reduction of tea time availability: 5 minutes from "steeping" to less than 30 seconds using blending.

Here is what I do to make a "water bottle" mixture for exercise. This uses bulk tea leaves (no tea bags, which are much more expensive).

- Place one to three tablespoons of raw dried Hibiscus flowers into a blender (mine is 64 ounce capacity).
- (optional) Add one to three tablespoons green tea leaves.
- Add a tablespoon of lemon or lime juice (to protect the antioxidants when blending).
- Add ice (optional) and water to three quarters of the capacity of the blender.
- (optional) If the sour bitter taste is an issue (I actually prefer it), add a date or date syrup to taste.

---

[426] Sleight, P., Yusuf, S., Pogue, J., Tsuyuki, R., Diaz, R., & Probstfield, J. (2001). Blood-pressure reduction and cardiovascular risk in HOPE study. *The Lancet,358*(9299), 2130-2131. doi:10.1016/s0140-6736(01) 07186-0.

- Blend mixture; up to 30 seconds.
- Remove blender container and strain directly into water bottles; will fill about three typical 24-ounce bottles.
- Can use one bottle now, refrigerate the others for later.

JUST SAY NO

Vital to vascular health is a healthy arterial endothelium, which is that single layer of cells found between the circulating blood and vascular smooth muscle cells discussed in Chapter 4. The endothelium controls blood pressure and arterial stiffness through controlling vascular tone.

The healthy endothelium maintains vascular homeostasis by synthesis of a wide range of molecules, including nitric oxide (abbreviated NO). Another source of nitric oxide is from the nitrate–nitrite–nitric oxide pathway[427]. In this pathway, about 25% of nitrate in the blood is actively absorbed by the salivary glands in the oral cavity and concentrated in the saliva. Anaerobic nitrate-reducing bacteria, located on the dorsal surface of the tongue, reduce that nitrate to nitrite[428]. The nitrite is absorbed into the bloodstream and becomes a source of nitric oxide for the endothelium[429].

---

[427] Webb, A. J., Patel, N., Loukogeorgakis, S., Okorie, M., Aboud, Z., Misra, S., . . . Ahluwalia, A. (2008). Acute Blood Pressure Lowering, Vaso-protective, and Antiplatelet Properties of Dietary Nitrate via Bioconversion to Nitrite.*Hypertension, 51*(3), 784-790. doi:10.1161/ hypertensionaha. 107.103523.

[428] Gladwin, M. T., Schechter, A. N., Kim-Shapiro, D. B., Patel, R. P., Hogg, N., Shiva, S., . . . Lundberg, J. O. (2005). The emerging biology of the nitrite anion. *Nature Chemical Biology, 1*(6), 308-314. doi:10.1038/ nchembio1105-308.

[429] Lundberg, J. O., & Govoni, M. (2004). Inorganic nitrate is a possible source for systemic generation of nitric oxide. *Free Radical Biology and Medicine, 37*(3), 395-400. doi:10.1016/ j.freeradbiomed. 2004.04.027.

Clinical studies have demonstrated lowering of blood pressure, improvement in endothelial function, and decreased arterial stiffness with nitrate intake. Vegetables are the primary sources of nitrate in the diet. Nitrate is absorbed effectively, with a bioavailability of 100%. Nitrate-rich vegetables include beetroot and beet greens, as well as other dark green leafy vegetables such as arugula and spinach (all more than 250 mg/100 g)[430].

> *Nitrate-rich vegetables such as dark green leafy vegetables and beetroot help lower blood pressure.*

While it has been established for a number of years now that fruits and vegetables assist with vascular health, this effect was thought to be primarily from the antioxidant properties such as that from carotenoids, but this has been largely disproven[431]. Instead, polyphenol flavonoids appear to be the phytonutrient more responsible for the effects on blood pressure and endothelial function along with dietary nitrates. While the molecular mechanisms by which flavonoids and nitrates reduce blood pressure are not completely understood, recent evidence suggests nitric oxide pathways[432].

---

[430] Santamaria, P. (2005). Nitrate in vegetables: Toxicity, content, intake and EC regulation. *Journal of the Science of Food and Agriculture J. Sci. Food Agric.,86*(1), 10-17. doi:10.1002/jsfa.2351.

[431] Bjelakovic, G., Nikolova, D., Gluud, L. L., Simonetti, R. G., & Gluud, C. (2007). Mortality in Randomized Trials of Antioxidant Supplements for Primary and Secondary Prevention. *Jama, 297*(8), 842. doi:10.1001/ jama.297.8.842.

[432] Bondonno, C. P., Croft, K. D., Ward, N., Considine, M. J., & Hodgson, J. M. (2015). Dietary flavonoids and nitrate: Effects on nitric oxide and vascular function. *Nutrition Reviews, 73*(4), 216-235. doi:10.1093/ nutrit/nuu014.

Beet it

Beetroot (Beta Vulgaris L.) contains biologically active phytochemicals including flavonoids and dietary nitrate. The antihypertensive effects of beetroot are attributed to the presence of inorganic nitrate in the plant. A randomized crossover study[433] of 250 ml/ day either of raw beet juice or 250 grams/ day of cooked beets showed a significant reduction in both systolic (average 7 mm Hg reduction) and diastolic (5 mm Hg reduction) blood pressure[434].

Not only would daily consumption of beet juice be effective for blood pressure control, it can be useful for enhancing athletic performance. A study of participants with peripheral artery disease showed a decrease in diastolic blood pressure 120 minutes after beetroot juice consumption[435]. Therefore, to assist with oxygenation capacity for aerobic sports or training, 8.5 fluid ounces (250 ml) of beet juice prior to the activity could have a significant effect[436].

---

[433] Asgary, S., Afshani, M. R., Sahebkar, A., Keshvari, M., Taheri, M., Jahanian, E., . . . Sarrafzadegan, N. (2016). Improvement of hypertension, endothelial function and systemic inflammation following short-term supplementation with red beet (Beta vulgaris L.) juice: A randomized crossover pilot study. *Journal of Human Hypertension, 30*(10), 627-632. doi:10.1038/jhh.2016.34.

[434] Cooked beets were slightly less effective by 1 mm Hg for both systolic and diastolic pressure, likely within experimental error.

[435] Kenjale, A. A., Ham, K. L., Stabler, T., Robbins, J. L., Johnson, J. L., Vanbruggen, M., . . . Allen, J. D. (2011). Dietary nitrate supplementation enhances exercise performance in peripheral arterial disease. *Journal of Applied Physiology, 110*(6), 1582-1591. doi:10.1152/ japplphysiol.00071.2011.

[436] I use Beet Performer Beet Juice 8.4 fluid ounces with B12; cost is $31.29 for a 12 pack.

There are home tests for monitoring of nitric oxide. For example, Berkeley Test makes saliva test strips analyzed colormetrically using an app and your smart phone camera.

As you shall read in Chapter 17 on blending, many daily nutritive requirements can be easily, conveniently, combined in in a food processing device that maximizes bioaccessibility.

INFLAMMATION

As we have previously reviewed in some detail, chronic subclinical inflammation has been recognized as a risk factor for a number of chronic diseases including cancer, vascular and neurodegenerative diseases. Among the components of a healthy non-inflammatory diet, whole grains, vegetables and fruits are all associated with lower inflammation[437] and studies have indicated diets containing animal products are pro-inflammatory, containing saturated fatty acids and trans-fatty acids.

Epidemiological evidence strongly suggests that long-term consumption of diets rich in plant polyphenols is capable of offering protection against the development of major chronic inflammatory and neurodegenerative diseases[438]. Polyphenol rich foods such as fruits, vegetables, dark chocolate[439] and

---

[437] Calder, P. C., Ahluwalia, N., Brouns, F., Buetler, T., Clement, K., Cunningham, K., . . . Winklhofer-Roob, B. M. (2011). Dietary factors and low-grade inflammation in relation to overweight and obesity. *British Journal of Nutrition, 106*(S3). doi:10.1017/s0007114511005460.

[438] Graf, B. A., Milbury, P. E., & Blumberg, J. B. (2005). Flavonols, Fla-vones, Flavanones, and Human Health: Epidemiological Evi-dence. *Journal of Medicinal Food, 8*(3), 281-290. doi:10.1089/ jmf.2005.8.281.

[439] di Giuseppe, R., Di Castelnuovo, A., Centritto, F., Zito, F., De Curtis, A., Costanzo, S., & ... Iacoviello, L. (2008). Regular Consumption of Dark Chocolate Is Associated with Low Serum Concentrations of C-Reactive

green tea, have been shown to reduce low-grade inflammation[440].

Polyphenols have been reported to reduce inflammation by acting as an antioxidant as well as by several additional mechanisms[441].

FRUITS AND VEGETABLES

Numerous studies have shown an inverse correlation between fruit and vegetable consumption and inflammation status. I advocate a whole-food varied-plant diet. A reason for the importance of "varied" is exhibited by the anti-inflammatory benefit of fruits and vegetables; the greater the variety, but not just quantity, the greater the benefit in terms of reducing the risk for diseases associated with chronic inflammation[442].

Protein in a Healthy Italian Population. *Journal Of Nutrition, 138*(10), 1939-1945.

[440] Scalbert, A., Manach, C., Morand, C., Rémésy, C., & Jiménez, L. (2005). Dietary Polyphenols and the Prevention of Diseases. *Critical Reviews in Food Science and Nutrition, 45*(4), 287-306. doi:10.1080/1040869059096.

[441] (a) attenuating endoplasmic reticulum stress signaling; (b) blocking pro-inflammatory cytokines or endotoxin-mediated kinases and transcription factors; (c) suppressing inflammatory or inducing metabolic gene expression via increasing histone deacetylase activity; (e) activating transcription factors that antagonize chronic inflammation: Pounis, G., Castelnuovo, A. D., Bonaccio, M., Costanzo, S., Persichillo, M., Krogh, V., . . . Iacoviello, L. (2015). Flavonoid and lignan intake in a Mediterranean population: Proposal for a holistic approach in polyphenol dietary analysis, the Moli-sani Study. *European Journal of Clinical Nutrition Eur J Clin Nutr, 70*(3), 338-345. doi:10.1038/ejcn.2015.178.

[442] Bhupathiraju, S. N., & Tucker, K. L. (2010). Greater variety in fruit and vegetable intake is associated with lower inflammation in Puerto Rican adults. *American Journal of Clinical Nutrition, 93*(1), 37-46. doi:10.3945/ajcn.2010.29913.

OMEGA-3

As previously discussed, polyunsaturated fatty acids antagonize and balance arachidonic acid metabolism and plays a key anti-inflammatory role; the omega-3s have other anti-inflammatory effects resulting from altered eicosanoid production.

Flaxseeds help to lower chronic inflammation

Plant sources of omega-3 fatty acids contain α-linolenic acid (ALA) and are found in flaxseeds, walnuts, pumpkin seeds, oatmeal, canola, and in lesser amounts in Brussels sprouts, kale, mint, parsley, spinach, and watercress.

Nuts

Epidemiologic and clinical trial evidence has demonstrated consistent benefits of tree nut consumption on modulating inflammation[443].

Nuts contain a variety of bioactive compounds: polyphenols, polyunsaturated fatty acids, fiber, and compounds called tocopherols and tocotrienols[444], all of which appear to contribute to the observed anti-inflammatory activities[445].

---

[443] Kris-etherton, P. M., Hu, F. B., Ros, E., & Sabaté6, J. (2008). The Role of Tree Nuts and Peanuts in the Prevention of Coronary Heart Disease: Multiple Potential Mechanisms. *Journal Of Nutrition, 138*(9), 1746S-1751S.

[444] Bolling, B. W., McKay, D. L., & Blumberg, J. B. (2010). The phytochemical composition and antioxidant actions of tree nuts. *Asia Pacific Journal Of Clinical Nutrition, 19*(1), 117-123.

[445] Bolling, B. W., Chen, C. O., McKay, D. L., & Blumberg, J. B. (2011). Tree nut phytochemicals: composition, antioxidant capacity, bioactivity, impact factors. A systematic review of almonds, Brazils, cashews, hazelnuts, macadamias, pecans, pine nuts, pistachios and walnuts. *Nutrition Research Reviews, 24*(2), 244-275. doi:10.1017/S095442241100014X.

Cocoa and chocolate

The health benefits of cocoa and dark chocolate, especially in their role of reducing the risk of vascular diseases, have been widely recognized[446]. Apparently, antioxidant activity is the major mechanism by which cocoa flavanols are responsible for the observed anti-inflammatory effects[447].

Tea

Tea drinking, particularly of green tea, has been inversely related to inflammation, owing to its main ingredient, catechin content, a compound belonging to the flavonoid family.

> *Tree nuts, cocoa, and tea have good anti-inflammatory properties.*

Fiber

Foods such as whole grains, fruits, vegetables, legumes, and nuts are rich sources of dietary fiber, including soluble and insoluble fiber.

The association of high dietary fiber intake and lower systemic inflammation is a more recent finding. In a review that included

---

[446] Cooper, K. A., Donovan, J. L., Waterhouse, A. L., & Williamson, G. (2007). Cocoa and health: A decade of research. *British Journal of Nutrition, 99*(01). doi:10.1017/s0007114507795296.

[447] Selmi, C., Cocchi, C. A., Lanfredini, M., Keen, C. L., & Gershwin, M. E. (2008). Chocolate at heart: The anti-inflammatory impact of cocoa flavanols. *Molecular Nutrition & Food Research Mol. Nutr. Food Res., 52*(11), 1340-1348. doi:10.1002/mnfr.200700435.

seven studies on the topic, significantly lower inflammatory markers were seen with increased fiber consumption[448].

However, the biological mechanism of anti-inflammatory effects of dietary fiber is largely unknown.

Recipe: Anti-inflammatory brownies

This recipe incorporates the anti-inflammatories flax, nuts, cacao, oats, and as an option and anti-inflammatory spices of your choice.

Ingredients

- 1/2 cup nut butter (eg, walnut or soy butter)
- 1 cup unsweetened cacao powder
- 1/2 cup ground cup flaxseed
- 1/2 cup oat flour
- 1 tsp baking powder
- 1/2 cup granulated erythritol or date crumbles
- 1/2 tsp vanilla extract
- 1/2 cup chocolate chips, 85% or better cacao content[449]
- (optional) add favorite anti-inflammatory spice (including cloves, cinnamon, turmeric, rosemary, ginger, sage, and thyme.)

Procedure

- Preheat oven to 325 F

---

[448] North, C. J., Venter, C. S., & Jerling, J. C. (2009). The effects of dietary fibre on C-reactive protein, an inflammation marker predicting cardiovascular disease. *European Journal Of Clinical Nutrition*, *63*(8), 921-933. doi:10.1038/ejcn.2009.8.

[449] For example, PASCHA Organic Dark Chocolate Baking Chips - 85% Cacao, Bitter-Sweet - 8.75 oz.

- In small saucepan over low heat, melt nut butter and cacao powder together until smooth. Set aside.
- In a medium bowl, whisk together flaxseed meal, oat flour, and baking powder. Set aside.
- In a large bowl, whisk together the granulated erythritol or date crumbles and vanilla extract. Whisk in melted chocolate mixture until smooth. Stir in the flaxseed meal mixture. Stir in chocolate chips.
- Bake 15 to 18 minutes, until top is just barely firm to the touch. Remove from oven and let cool, then cut into sections.

OXIDATIVE STRESS

Oxidative stress and inflammation are closely linked to various chronic diseases, as explored in Chapter 6, and anti-oxidants play a pivotal role. Oxidative damage and inflammatory processes initiate the first stage of vascular disease resulting from the interaction of excess reactive free radicals with cell structures.

Also detailed in Chapter 6 was the etiologic influence of oxidative stress on mental disorders from a number of different mechanisms.

Which plants have the highest anti-oxidant content?

All plants have antioxidants, but some much more than others. Keeping in mind the protective function of antioxidants in plants for the safety of the plants themselves, it makes sense to consider those plants (or plant parts) having the most surface-toward-the-sun to volume ratio. The winners in this regard are leaves – and the darker the better as the sun's energy is absorbed into the leaf more fully the darker it is.

Beginning in 1980, a semi-quantitative food frequency questionnaire was administered by researchers at Harvard Medical School every four years to the more than 15,000 Nurses' Health Study participants[450]. In 1995–2001, they began measuring cognitive function in participants aged 70 years or older. Follow-up assessments were conducted twice, at two-year intervals. Their conclusion was:

> *"We found that higher consumption of berries and anthocyanidins, as well as total flavonoids, is associated with a slower progression of cognitive decline in older women. These findings potentially have substantial public health implications, as increasing berry intake represents a fairly simple dietary modification to test in older adults for maintaining cognition."*

That study focused on blueberries and strawberries – the fruit kernels; it is interesting to note that the anthocyanin content of the leaves of these fruits is about ten times higher than the

Certain grapes, berries and eggplant have high concentrations of an effective type of antioxidant.

[450] Devore, E. E., Kang, J. H., Breteler, M. M., & Grodstein, F. (2012). Dietary intakes of berries and flavonoids in relation to cognitive decline. *Annals of Neurology Ann Neurol.*, 72(1), 135-143. doi:10.1002/ana.23594.

berries[451] [452]. As for "total flavonoids", tea (green leaves) contained the most – by a substantial margin.

Considering commonly available fruits, the following table lists those with higher anthocyanin content[453] [454] [455] [456] [457] [458]:

---

[451] Fanning, K., Edwards, D., Netzel, M., Stanley, R., Netzel, G., Russell, D., & Topp, B. (2013). Increasing Anthocyanin Content In Queen Garnet Plum And Correlations With In-Field Measures. *Acta Hortic. Acta Horticulturae*, (985), 97-104. doi:10.17660/actahortic.2013.985.12.

[452] Vyas, P; Kalidindi, S; Chibrikova, L; et al. (2013). "Chemical analysis and effect of blueberry and lingonberry fruits and leaves against glutamate-mediated excitotoxicity". *Journal of Agricultural and Food Chemistry* 61 (32): 7769–76.

[453] Siriwoharn T; Wrolstad RE; Finn CE; et al. (December 2004). "Influence of cultivar, maturity, and sampling on blackberry (Rubus L. Hybrids) anthocyanins, polyphenolics, and antioxidant properties". *Journal of Agricultural and Food Chemistry* 52 (26): 8021–30.

[454] Wada L; Ou B (June 2002). "Antioxidant activity and phenolic content of Oregon caneberries". *Journal of Agricultural and Food Chemistry* 50 (12): 3495–500.

[455] Hosseinian FS; Beta T (December 2007). "Saskatoon and wild blueberries have higher anthocyanin contents than other Manitoba berries". *Journal of Agricultural and Food Chemistry* **55** (26): 10832–8.

[456] Wu X; Beecher GR; Holden JM; et al. (November 2006). "Concentrations of anthocyanins in common foods in the United States and estimation of normal consumption". *Journal of Agricultural and Food Chemistry* 54 (11): 4069–75.

[457] *Fanning K; Edwards D; Netzel M; et al. (November 2013). "Increasing anthocyanin content in Queen Garnet plum and correlations with in-field measures". Acta Horticulturae 985: 97–104.*

[458] Muñoz-Espada, A. C.; Wood, K. V.; Bordelon, B.; et al. (2004). "Anthocyanin Quantification and Radical Scavenging Capacity of Concord, Norton, and Marechal Foch Grapes and Wines". *Journal of Agricultural and Food Chemistry* 52 (22): 6779–86.

Table 5 Anthocyanin Antioxidant Properties for Select Fruit

Fruit	Anthocyanin mg/100 g
Norton grape	888
Eggplant	750
Black raspberry	589
Wild blueberry	558
Red raspberry	365
Blackberry	317
Concord grape	326
Plum	277
Cherry	122

TOTAL ANTIOXIDANT CONTENT

The most comprehensive analysis of the antioxidant content of over 3000 foods was performed at the University of Oslo[459]. The results indicate that there are several thousand-fold differences in antioxidant content of foods. Spices and herbs are the most antioxidant-rich. Berries, fruits, nuts, chocolate, and select vegetables also are rich in antioxidants. We shall list the antioxidant content of a number of foods in food groups (the unit of concentration is milli-moles per 100 gram of whole food), starting with beverages.

---

[459] Carlsen, M. H., Halvorsen, B. L., Holte, K., Bøhn, S. K., Dragland, S., Sampson, L., . . . Blomhoff, R. (2010). The total antioxidant content of more than 3100 foods, beverages, spices, herbs and supplements used worldwide. Nutrition Journal Nutr J, 9(1). doi:10.1186/1475-2891-9-3; for a full listing of all results, see: http://www.biomedcentral.com/ content/supplementary/1475-2891-9-3-S1.pdf.

Beverages

The highest antioxidant values in this category were found among the unprocessed tea leaves and coffee beans. The best way to consume tea leaves and coffee beans is to eat them. The data in the Oslo study is somewhat misleading in that dry leaves and beans are compared to the drink after adding hot water. However, only consuming the water soluble nutrients undoubtedly loses the full extent of the available nutrients.

Other antioxidant rich beverages include various red wines, which have an antioxidant content of 1.78 to 3.66 mmol/100 g. Beer has a significant amount of antioxidants. Samichclaus beer, touted as the strongest beer in the world and brewed once per year on "Santa Claus Day" has the maximum antioxidant content of all beers. Cola and energy drinks effectively have no antioxidants.

Figure 14 Antioxidant Properties of Select Beverages

Beverage	Antioxidant, mmol/100 g
Tea, green, dry	24.31
Coffee beans, dark roasted	22.29
Coffee, Arabica strong roasting, filter brewed	2.69
Wine, red, Chianti	2.68
Tea, green, Earl Grey, prepared	1.43
Samichlaus Bier	0.46
Coca-Cola	0.05
Red Bull energy drink	0

Meat and dairy products

The meat and dairy categories were very low in antioxidant content and will not be further detailed here.

Fruit

The average antioxidant content of berries is relatively high, the highest being dried amla (Indian gooseberry) at 261.5 mmol/100 g. Amla is extremely bitter, so I swallow a 250 mg capsule of the whole dried berry (plus 350 mg of the stem) each day for a cost of less than 25 cents.

> *Fruits, like berries, have high antioxidant content.*

The skin of citrus fruits is high in antioxidants, higher than the fruit flesh. Apples and bananas are relatively low in antioxidants; this explains the darkening of these fruits once exposed to air.

Figure 15 Antioxidant Content of Select Fruits

Fruit	Antioxidant, mmol/100 g
Amla berries, dried	261.53
Blackberries, wild	6.14
Blackberries, cultivated	4.13
Lemon Skin	2.74
Raspberries, cultivated	2.33
Strawberries, cultivated	2.16
Blueberries, cultivated	1.85
Lemon	1.02
Grapes, blue	0.9
Lime	0.47
Apples, red delicious	0.4

Vegetables

In the table below, are listed the anti-oxidant content of a few vegetables.

Examples of antioxidant rich vegetables are artichokes, curly kale, colored bell peppers, red cabbage and beetroot.

Figure 16 Antioxidant Properties of Select Vegetables

Vegetable	Antioxidant, mmol/100 g
Artichoke, boiled	3.89
Cauliflower, blue, cooked	3.52
Kale, curly	2.68
Bell pepper (red, yellow, orange)	1.8
Cabbage, red	1.78
Beetroot	1.68
Spinach	0.89
Leaves of sweet potato plant	0.48
Garlic	0.22
Sweet potato	0.08
Carrots	0.03

Nuts and seeds

In the nuts and seeds category, antioxidant contents for nuts with the pellicle, or thin skin surrounding the nut, are significant for walnuts and less so for almonds; however, typical commercially prepared nuts do not have the bitter pellicle. Nevertheless, walnuts even without the pellicle have significant antioxidant content. Peanuts, actually a legume, are a fair source of antioxidants, as are pistachios. Flaxseeds and Brazil nuts have some antioxidant value as well.

Figure 17 Antioxidant Content of Select Nuts and Seeds

Nuts and Seeds	Antioxidant, mmol/100 g
Walnuts, with pellice	14.29
Peanuts, roasted in shell	1.97
Walnuts, without pellice	1.81
Pistachios	1.43
Flaxseeds	0.8
Brazil nuts	0.66
Almonds with pellice	0.53
Almonds without pellice	0.13

St. John's wort

Preparations with standardized extracts of St. John's wort, for example available in Germany by prescription, are well established for the treatment of depressive disorders of mild-to-medium severity[460]. Various placebo-controlled clinical trials have confirmed its antidepressant potency, which is comparable to synthetic antidepressants, such as imipramine or sertraline. Side effects are usually less pronounced and less severe compared to standard antidepressants, although there is a known inhibition of liver enzymes and therefore interactions with various medications. However, as this plant is not FDA approved in the United States for use as an antidepressant, doses are not standardized. This plant has

---

[460] Linde, K., Mulrow, C., Berner, M., & Egger, M. (2005). St John's Wort for depression. *Cochrane Database of Systematic Reviews Reviews.* doi:10.1002/14651858.cd000448.pub2.

excellent antioxidant properties but the mechanism of activity as an antidepressant is unknown.

Saffron

Another one of the antioxidant-rich spices is saffron. Saffron is a spice derived from the flower stigma of Crocus sativus. Although used for thousands of years in traditional medicine as an anticonvulsive, analgesic and aphrodisiac, among other uses[461], modern pharmacological studies have demonstrated that extracts of

> *Saffron appears to have promise as an anti-depressant.*

saffron stigmas have anticancer, anti-inflammatory, antioxidant and antiplatelet effects – and now antidepressant effects[462].

Saffron has now undergone a number of trials examining its antidepressant effects and, in a recent meta-analysis, was confirmed to be effective for the treatment of major depression.

Recent comprehensive and statistically significant meta-analyses confirmed saffron as an efficacious treatment of depression[463].

---

[461] Hosseinzadeh, H., & Nassiri-Asl, M. (2012). Avicenna's (Ibn Sina) the Canon of Medicine and Saffron (Crocus sativus): A Review. *Phytother. Res. Phytotherapy Research, 27*(4), 475-483. doi:10.1002/ptr.484.

[462] Wang, Y., Han, T., Zhu, Y., Zheng, C., Ming, Q., Rahman, K., & Qin, L. (2009). Antidepressant properties of bioactive fractions from the extract of Crocus sativus L. *Journal of Natural Medicines J Nat Med, 64*(1), 24-30. doi:10.1007/s11418-009-0360-6.

[463] Hausenblas, H. A., Saha, D., Dubyak, P. J., & Anton, S. D. (2013). Saffron (Crocus sativus L.) and major depressive disorder: A meta-analysis of randomized clinical trials. *Journal of Integrative Medicine, 11*(6), 377-383. doi:10.3736/jintegrmed2013056.

Given the many bioactive constituents contained in saffron, it likely has several antidepressant mechanisms of action, including its antioxidant, anti-inflammatory, serotonergic, hypothalamus-pituitary-adrenal axis modulation and neuro-protective effects. The side effect profile is superior to those of the commercial antidepressants reviewed, with the typical dose of saffron being 30 mg twice per day[464]. Toxicity at higher doses appears to be quite low[465].

For example, in a double-blind randomized clinical trial, saffron (this study used saffron at 30 mg per day, costing about 20 cents per dose[466]) was equally effective in treating mild to moderate depression as the oft-compared earliest effective antidepressant that started the anti-depressant pharmacological revolution, namely imipramine[467]. See Chapter 14 for more information on saffron.

[464] Lopresti, A. L., & Drummond, P. D. (2014). Saffron (Crocus sativus) for depression: a systematic review of clinical studies and examination of underlying antidepressant mechanisms of action.*Human Psychopharmacology: Clinical & Experimental, 29*(6), 517-527. doi:10.1002/hup.2434

[465] Melnyk, J. P., Wang, S., & Marcone, M. F. (2010). Chemical and biological properties of the world's most expensive spice: Saffron. *Food Research International, 43*(8), 1981-1989. doi:10.1016/ j.foodres.2010.07.033.

[466] For example, Kiva Gourmet, Spanish Saffron, Premium-grade 3 gram bottle costs $20.99 delivered through Amazon Prime.

[467] Akhondzadeh, S. (n.d.). Comparison of Crocus sativus L. and imipramine in the treatment of mild to moderate depression: A pilot double-blind randomised trial. *Http://isrctn.org/.* doi:10.1186/ isrctn45683816.

Spices and Herbs

Spices and herbs have very high antioxidant content. Sorted by antioxidant content, cloves have the highest mean antioxidant value by far, followed by mint, St. John's wort, oregano, saffron and sage, all dried and ground.

Refer to the table below for relative concentrations of antioxidants in spices and herbs.

Figure 18 Antioxidant Contents of Select Herbs and Spices

Spices and Herbs	Antioxidant, mmol/100 g
Clove, dried, ground (average)	300
Mint, green, leaves, dried	142.58
St. John's wort, flower and leaves, dried	72.16
Oregano, dried (average)	70
Saffron, dried, ground (average)	50
Sage, leaves, dried	39.36
Yarrow, flower and leaves, dried	31.66
Nutmeg, dried, ground (average)	30
Dandelion, leaves, dried	21.07
Cinnamon, dried, ground	17.65
Dill, dried (average)	15
Dandelion, flower, dried	12.72
Chili, dried, ground	12.21
Turmeric, dried, ground (average)	12
Cumin, dried, ground	10.31
Curry, powder	9.98
Pepper, black, dried (average)	7
Cayenne pepper, dried	5.38
Basil, fresh	0.82

Chocolate

Various types of chocolate were analyzed, from milk chocolate to dark chocolate to baking cocoa. The variation of antioxidant content in chocolate ranged from 0.23 in white chocolate to 14.98 mmol/100 g in one individual dark chocolate sample. Mean antioxidant content increased with increasing cocoa content in the chocolate product. Chocolate with cocoa contents of 24-30%, 40-65% and 70-99% had mean antioxidant contents of 1.8, 7.2 and 10.9 mmol/100 g, respectively.

The conclusion of the scientists at the University of Oslo who provided this vast number of antioxidant measurements in food was:

> *"Antioxidant-rich foods originate from the plant kingdom while meat, fish and other foods from the animal kingdom are low in antioxidants. Diets comprised mainly of animal-based foods are thus low in antioxidant content while diets based mainly on a variety of plant-based foods are antioxidant rich, due to the thousands of bioactive antioxidant phytochemicals found in plants..."*

CHAPTER 14

Psychotropic Nutraceutics

"Unless someone like you cares a whole lot, nothing is going to get better. It's not."

The Lorax - Dr. Seuss

HAPPY MEALS

In the last chapter, each currently recognized pathophysiologic condition related to cognitive, emotional, and behavioral decline was summarized with indications on how to prevent or reverse each condition using dietary and other interventions.

In earlier chapters, these etiologic mechanisms affecting our mental health were detailed, with extensive references for those wishing to have a deeper understanding.

With the hope that a degree of credibility has been established on the food-mood link, this chapter will expand and summarize what you can do for your mind-body emphasizing specific foods within the whole-food varied-plant dietary pattern.

GREEN LEAFY VEGETABLES

If you were stranded on a desert island and could have only one type of food, what would it be? You would probably choose a type of fruit — coconuts would be a fun choice — but a green leafy vegetable like kale would be superior in nutrients, important if your tenure on the island is prolonged.

> *Try to include greens with every meal. It's easiest to include in a blended combo with fruit but can be mashed or chopped and added to most any meal.*

Besides pretty much covering the spectrum of important nutrients, greens specifically have omega-3s, an excellent omega 6 to 3 ratio, and soluble fibers for vascular health. They are generally high in nitrates for blood pressure control.

Greens are anti-inflammatory, partly as a result of their alkalinity, omega-3, and fiber content. They are also rich in antioxidants. Teas and herbs are usually green leaves, too, but shall be explored separately.

GREEN TEA

Tea is the most consumed beverage in the world. It comes from an evergreen called *Camellia sinensis*. "Green" tea merely refers to the natural state of the tea plant; in the United States, the preference is for "black" tea, a less healthy oxidized version.

Green tea offers incredible health benefits but is consumed mainly for its psychoactive ingredients: caffeine and L-theanine, or just theanine[468]. The stimulating effect of caffeine is modulated by the calming effect of theanine.

When theanine is consumed, it peaks in the serum within an hour[469] and is at its maximum level in the brain within 5 hours, gradually disappears from the liver, kidney, and brain within 24 hours[470].

Theanine readily crosses the blood–brain barrier where it exerts a variety of neurophysiological and pharmacological effects. Its most well-documented effect has been its apparent anxiolytic and calming effect due to its up regulation of inhibitory neurotransmitters; however, there is also evidence of increases of the neurotransmitters serotonin and dopamine in selected areas such as the midbrain[471].

Tea is very rich in polyphenols, accounting for up to 30% of the dry weight of tea. Tea has positive effects on cognitive functioning beyond the stimulating effect from caffeine

---

[468] Here use of the name "theanine" without a "L-" prefix is understood to imply the L-enantiomer, which is the form found in fresh teas and in some, but not all dietary supplements.

[469] Unno, T., Suzuki, Y., Kakuda, T., Hayakawa, T., & Tsuge, H. (1999). Metabolism of Theanine, γ-Glutamylethylamide, in Rats. *J. Agric. Food Chem. Journal of Agricultural and Food Chemistry, 47*(4), 1593-1596. doi:10.1021/jf981113t.

[470] Terashima, T., Takido, J., & Yokogoshi, H. (1999). Time-dependent Changes of Amino Acids in the Serum, Liver, Brain and Urine of Rats Administered with Theanine. *Bioscience, Biotechnology, and Biochemistry, 63*(4), 615-618. doi:10.1271/bbb.63.615.

[471] Lardner, A. L. (2013). Neurobiological effects of the green tea constituent theanine and its potential role in the treatment of psychiatric and neurodegenerative disorders. *Nutritional Neuroscience, 17*(4), 145-155. doi:10.1179/1476830513y.0000000079.

through possibly enhancing short-term plasticity in the pare-frontal brain areas.

Investigations have found that higher consumption of green tea led to a lower prevalence of depressive symptoms in elderly Japanese individuals[472]. Another study indicated the mechanism may involve inhibition of the hypothalamic-pituitary-adrenal (HPA) axis[473]. Some research indicates that the anhedonia associated with clinical depression is particularly improved with green tea consumption.[474]

L-theanine

Emerging studies also demonstrate a promising role for theanine in augmentation therapy for schizophrenia. Some early studies are beginning to examine a putative role in attention deficit hyperactivity disorder, and in other psychiatric disorders such as anxiety disorders, panic disorder, and obsessive compulsive disorder (OCD)[475].

Theanine also elicits improvements in cognitive function including learning and memory. One study investigated the

---

[472] Buckley, P. (2011). Green tea consumption is associated with depressive symptoms in the elderly. *Yearbook of Psychiatry and Applied Mental Health,2011*, 377-379. doi:10.1016/s0084-3970(10)79364-6.

[473] Zhu, W., Shi, H., Wei, Y., Wang, S., Sun, C., Ding, Z., & Lu, L. (2012). Green tea polyphenols produce antidepressant-like effects in adult mice. *Pharmacological Research, 65*(1), 74-80. doi:10.1016/j.phrs.2011.09.007.

[474] Qiangye, Z., Hongchao, Y., Jian, W., Aiwu, L., Wentong, Z., Xinhai, C., & Kelai, W. (2013). Effect of green tea on reward learning in healthy individuals: a randomized, double-blind, placebo-controlled pilot study. *Nutrition Journal,12*(1), 1-7. doi:10.1186/1475-2891-12-84.

[475] Lardner, A. L. (2013). Neurobiological effects of the green tea constituent theanine and its potential role in the treatment of psychiatric and neurodegenerative disorders. *Nutritional Neuroscience, 17*(4), 145-155. doi:10.1179/1476830513y.0000000079.

effects of 47.5 mg theanine daily on cognitive function in the elderly and reported significantly lower decline than in controls[476]. Another study reported lower incidences of cognitive impairments in human subjects ingesting theanine in the form of two or more cups of green tea daily.

It has also recently been shown to increase levels of brain-derived neurotrophic factor. An increasing number of studies demonstrate neuroprotective effects following cerebral infarct and injury, although the exact molecular mechanisms remain to be fully elucidated[477].

> *A cup or two of green tea is recommended every day; alternatively a heaping tablespoon of bulk green tea is excellent in a morning smoothie.*

In addition to its ability to alter neurotransmitter activity, theanine has also been found to significantly increase alpha brain wave activity. Alpha brain wave activity in humans is indicative of wakeful relaxation, increased creativity, better performance under stress, and improved learning and concentration, as well as decreased anxiety[478]. So theanine appears to exert a positive role in the focusing of selective attention and reduction of distracting stimuli by means of its effects on alpha brain wave activity. Increases in alpha brain

---

[476] Kakuda, T. (2011). Neuroprotective effects of theanine and its preventive effects on cognitive dysfunction. *Pharmacological Research, 64*(2), 162-168. doi:10.1016/j.phrs.2011.03.010.

[477] Lardner, A. L. (2013). Neurobiological effects of the green tea constituent theanine and its potential role in the treatment of psychiatric and neurodegenerative disorders. *Nutritional Neuroscience, 17*(4), 145-155. doi:10.1179/1476830513y.0000000079.

[478] Eschenauer, G. (2006). Pharmacology and therapeutic uses of theanine. *American Journal of Health-System Pharmacy, 63*(1), 26-30. doi:10.2146/ajhp050148.

wave activity are in the occipital, parietal and frontal areas following consumption of 50–250 mg theanine.

A "pharmaceutical composition" of theanine has been proposed by Taiyo Kagaku Company of Japan as a patent (US Patent Application 20040171624; Japanese Patent Application 2001-253740), claiming:

> *"A pharmaceutical composition for treating or preventing mood disorders, comprising theanine. A food or beverage for ameliorating or preventing mood disorders, comprising theanine. The pharmaceutical composition and the food and beverage are safe and have a significant suppressive effect on the depression in a mood disorder."*

FRUITS

Of the individual dietary risk factors for death, the Global Burden of Disease study[479] found that the largest attributable burden in 2010 was associated with *diets low in fruits* (4.9 million deaths).

> *Remember that low fruit intake is the leading dietary cause of death in the world. Eat 3 servings per day (about 3 cups chopped equivalent; include berries).*

---

[479] S. Lim S, Vos T, Blyth F, et al. A comparative risk assessment of burden of disease and injury attributable to 67 risk factors and risk factor clusters in 21 regions, 1990-2010: a systematic analysis for the Global Burden of Disease Study 2010. Lancet [serial online]. December 15, 2012;380(9859):2224-2260. Available from: Academic Search Com-plete, Ipswich, MA. Accessed October 2, 2016.

Fruits have significant fiber, particularly soluble fiber, assisting cholesterol control and therefore reducing vascular disease risk.

But fruits, particularly *berries*, are antioxidant champions. I detailed in Chapter 6 the etiologic influence of oxidative stress on mental disorders from a number of different mechanisms.

There is such a wonderful variety of fruits and with their sweet taste, they are usually great eaten alone or in combination with other more bitter or bland foods.

Fruits make terrific snacks throughout the day.

NUTS AND SEEDS

Recall the favorable effect of tree nuts on cholesterol, likely as a result of fiber (about 25% soluble), micronutrients such as vitamins E and C, folic acid, copper, magnesium, selenium, plant sterols, and phenolic components.

Consumption of 50 – 100 g/ day of nuts (about a heaping palm-full or half a cup), especially almonds, Brazil, peanuts, pecans, or walnuts[480], significantly lowers LDL-cholesterol.

Nuts are also a great snack and in combination with other foods, adds crunch, flavor, and fat content which is important for absorption of fat soluble nutrients. Toasted nuts are okay but no salted nuts, please.

---

[480] I like "Food To Live Mixed Raw Nuts" (Cashews, Brazil Nuts, Walnuts, Almonds).

SEEDS

Seeds are a good food source because they contain the nutrients necessary for the plant's initial growth, including many healthy fats such as omega-3s.

In fact, the majority of foods consumed by human beings are seed-based, including cereals, legumes (beans, peas, lentils) and even nuts (technically a fruit with a hard shell and a single seed in most cases).

But there is one type of seed that I wish to emphasize beyond all else – perhaps the most important single food suggested by this book: flaxseed.

Flaxseed

You have noticed by now that flaxseed has been mentioned frequently. It helps lower cholesterol, lowers blood pressure, is anti-inflammatory, has good anti-oxidants, and fiber. It is the single most neuroprotective food; oh yes, then there is the omega-3 content.

There is no doubt that this food is an excellent source of essential omega-3 fats in the form of alpha-linolenic acid, the basic building block to other omega-3s - eicosapentaenoic acid and docosahexaenoic acid. We have detailed that omega-3, and a proper omega-3 to omega-6 ratio, is important in mental wellness and recovery from psychiatric disorders.

But flaxseed offers more than just the ideal omega-3 source; it contains many polyphenolic compounds such as phenolic acids[481], flavonoids and lignans along with vitamins C and E[482].

---

[481] Oomah, B. D., Kenaschuk, E. O., & Mazza, G. (1995). Phenolic Acids in Flaxseed. J. Agric. Food Chem. Journal of Agricultural and Food Chemistry, 43(8), 2016-2019. doi:10.1021/jf00056a011.

One study found that flaxseed significantly decreased chronic stress (cortisol) levels, indicating a possible synergistic effect between omega-3 fatty acid and polyphenols[483]. Other components such as a flaxseed lignan (a phytoestrogen compound called secoisolariciresinol) has been shown to have possible applications in post-menopausal depression[484].

Studies of flaxseed oil supplementation have indicated a good tolerance even in the pediatric population where one study indicated its effectiveness in child bipolar disorder[485].

I recommend a daily intake of one to three tablespoons of ground flax, each tablespoon of which contains about 30 calories, 2.5 grams fat, 2 grams fiber, and 1.5 grams protein[486]. Be sure to grind the flaxseeds as the fine seeds with their hard shell will likely just pass on through the gut otherwise. Flaxseeds can be ground in a coffee bean grinder and the

---

[482] Bidlack, W. W. (1999). Functional Foods: Biochemical and Processing Aspects, G. Mazza, ed. Lancaster, PA: Technomic Publishing Co., Inc., 437 pp, 1998. Journal of the American College of Nutrition, 18(6), 640-641. doi:10.1080/07315724.1999.10718899.

[483] Naveen, S., Siddalingaswamy, M., Singsit, D., & Khanum, F. (2013). Anti-depressive effect of polyphenols and omega-3 fatty acid from pomegranate peel and flax seed in mice exposed to chronic mild stress. Psychiatry Clin Neurosci Psychiatry and Clinical Neurosciences, 67(7), 501-508. doi:10.1111/pcn.12100.

[484] Wang, Y., Xu, Z., Yang, D., Yao, H., Ku, B., Ma, X., . . . Cai, S. (2012). The antidepressant effect of secoisolariciresinol, a lignan-type phytoestrogen constituent of flaxseed, on ovariectomized mice. Journal of Natural Medicines,67(1), 222-227. doi:10.1007/s11418-012-0655-x.

[485] Gracious, B. L., Chirieac, M. C., Costescu, S., Finucane, T. L., Youngstrom, E. A., & Hibbeln, J. R. (2010). Randomized, placebo-controlled trial of flax oil in pediatric bipolar disorder. Bipolar Disorders, 12(2), 142-154. doi:10.1111/j.1399-5618.2010.00799.x.

[486] A very convenient way to have ground flax ready to serve is provided by Carrington Farms Organic Ground Milled Flax Seeds, two tablespoon packets sealed and lasting without refrigeration about one year.

ground powder added to grains, salads, beans – practically any dish for a little texture.

Note that the shelf life of the oily seeds is limited unless kept in an airtight container in the fridge or freezer. Ground flaxseeds or flax meal should be kept in the freezer; at room temperature and exposed to air, use the ground seeds within one week. Smell the flax – if it has a strong odor such as fishy smell, it may be rancid. A taste test should reveal a mild nutty flavor – if bitter or sour that also may be a signal that it is rancid.

> *Flaxseeds are the single most important food for brain health. Consume 1 – 3 tablespoons per day. Every day.*

For these reasons, chia seeds, rich in antioxidants and omega-3 PUFAs may be preferable to some.

The following are some alternative ways to get your daily flax fix.

Flax four ways

1. Blended flax

My daily routine includes a blended drink of a number of nutrient-dense whole foods; this includes at least one tablespoon of flaxseed. A high-speed blender will easily grind flaxseeds through a combination of shear force and cavitation.

2. Oatmeal flax

Alternatively, flax can be introduced to oatmeal. See the portfolio diet oatmeal recipe in Chapter 13. One or two tablespoons of ground flaxseeds are mixed into the oatmeal.

3. Bake with Flaxseeds.

Take any basic bread product recipe and add one or more tablespoons of ground flaxseed. Nutrient content of flaxseed is acceptably stable at baking temperatures.

4. Flax crackers

Another favorite cooking method at low temperature is dehydration (Chapter 16). The flaxseeds crisped will be easier to crush while chewing to release the nutrients within, although you could try to mix in ground flax seeds as well.

Recipe: Flax Craxs

This recipe uses a dehydrator, discussed in Chapter 16.

Ingredients

- 1 cup (150g) flaxseed
- ¾ cup (190ml) water
- 3 tsp (15ml) Braggs soy sauce
- 3 tsp (15 ml) pure organic date syrup
- ½ tsp onion powder
- ½ tsp garlic powder

Instructions

- Place the whole (and optional ground) flaxseed and the rest of the mixture into a container and mix well.
- Stir or let sit until thickened.
- Place on solid dehydrator trays at 125 F for at least 3 hours.

- For extra crispy crackers, allow hydration all day or overnight.

Produces a great aroma while cooking. On holidays, I have made wreaths of flax crackers, a perfect shape for the circular trays of most dehydrators.

Other shapes can be made using cookie cutters. Cutting before too crisp is recommended.

This recipe make great tasting crackers, but of course one could slather with fruit, nut butter, hummus – many possibilities.

WHOLE GRAIN

Certain wild cereals, or grasses, contain edible components in their grain, botanically a type of fruit. Grains are small, hard, dry seeds, with or without attached hulls.

Some argue that from an evolutionary standpoint, grains are a relatively new addition to our diets and therefore should be excluded.

Undoubtedly grains have existed for many millennia, but the problem with harvesting had been that first of all these grains must be separated from the inedible grasses, requiring some winnowing process. Secondly, the wild grains usually shatter when ripe, dispersing the seeds, making collection difficult. Then the tiny hard grains would have to be further processed to avail digestion. Thus, patches of such grains in the wild may not have been favored by hominids until at least primitive hand tools were used and present near sites of grain-containing grasses.

Nevertheless, grains were apparently consumed well before animal domestication 10,000 years ago.

For example, a large amount of starch granules has been found on the surfaces of Middle Stone Age stone tools from Mozambique, showing that early Homo sapiens relied on grass seeds starting at least 105,000 years ago, including those of sorghum grasses[487]. That's more than 5000 generations ago.

Of course if one has celiac disease, gluten intolerance, a food allergy or sensitivity to grains, grains should be avoided.

GRAINS FOR BRAINS (AS WELL AS OTHER ORGANS)

Whole grain includes dark bread, whole-grain breakfast cereal, popcorn, oats, bran, brown rice, bran, and many other examples.

Whole-grain foods contain fiber, vitamins, magnesium and other minerals, phenolic compounds and other phytonutrients[488], which may have favorable effects on health by lowering serum lipids and blood pressure, improving glucose levels, insulin metabolism and endothelial function, as well as alleviating oxidative stress and inflammation.

A meta-analysis of 15 cohort studies with nearly a half million participants revealed that whole grain intake was associated with a reduced risk of vascular disease[489].

---

[487] Mercader, J. (2009), Mozambican Grass Seed Consumption During the Middle Stone Age, Science, 326.

[488] Anderson, J. W. (2003). Whole grains protect against atherosclerotic cardiovascular disease. *Proceedings of the Nutrition Society, 62*(01), 135-142. doi:10.1079/pns2002222.

[489] Tang, G., Wang, D., Long, J., Yang, F., & Si, L. (2015). Meta-Analysis of the Association Between Whole Grain Intake and Coronary Heart Disease Risk. *The American Journal of Cardiology, 115*(5), 625-629.

There is an association between dietary whole grain intake and mortality; two large prospective studies of more than one hundred thousand participants indicated a significant life extension independent of other dietary and lifestyle factors[490].

Eat at least one half cup of whole grains per day, such as one cup of oats and/ or one slice of whole grain bread.

The effect was pronounced up to one-half serving per day after which there was a leveling off. This is shown in the figure below, taken from the Wu et al. aforementioned article, where the mortality risk is plotted against servings of whole grain.

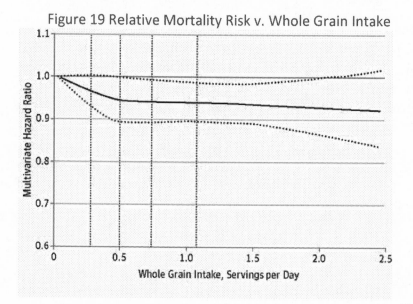

Figure 19 Relative Mortality Risk v. Whole Grain Intake

---

[490] Wu, H., Flint, A. J., Qi, Q., Dam, R. M., Sampson, L. A., Rimm, E. B., . . . Sun, Q. (2015). Association Between Dietary Whole Grain Intake and Risk of Mortality.*JAMA Internal Medicine JAMA Intern Med, 175*(3), 373.

NUTRITIONAL YEAST

Nutritional yeast has a nutty, cheesy flavor and is often used to emulate cheese, thicken sauces and dressings, and to provide an additional boost of nutrients, particularly B vitamins, folates, thiamine, riboflavin, niacin, selenium and zinc. It is a complete source of essential amino acids.

Impressive research exists that supports a positive effect of nutritional yeast on stress and related immune function resulting, for example, in a decrease for the susceptibility to the common cold[491]. Beta glucan fiber, found in baker's, brewer's and nutritional yeast, helps to maintain our body's defense against pathogens. And this is extended to improvement in mood states, related to immune vitality and emotional vitality[492].

> *Keep a container of nutritional yeast on your countertop and regularly, even daily, use about one heaping tablespoon (4 grams) on a variety of foods.*

For endurance athletes who place significant stress on their bodies, regular ingestion of this substance is recommended.

---

[491] Auinger, A., Riede, L., Bothe, G., Busch, R., & Gruenwald, J. (2013). Yeast (1,3)-(1,6)-beta-glucan helps to maintain the body's defence against pathogens: A double-blind, randomized, placebo-controlled, multicentric study in healthy subjects. *European Journal of Nutrition, 52*(8), 1913-1918. doi:10.1007/s00394-013-0492-z.

[492] Talbott, S. M., & Talbott, J. A. (2012). Baker's Yeast Beta-Glucan Supplement Reduces Upper Respiratory Symptoms and Improves Mood State in Stressed Women. *Journal of the American College of Nutrition, 31*(4), 295-300. doi:10.1080/07315724.2012.10720441.

COCOA

Foods and beverages made with beans from the Theobroma cacao tree have been consumed by humans for over 5000 years, in pre-Colombian cultures along the Yucatan, including the Mayans[493].

Cocoa is the dried and fully fermented fatty seed of the fruit of the cocoa tree, native to the Americas. Cocoa liquor is the paste made from ground, roasted, shelled, and fermented cocoa beans, called nibs. It contains both nonfat cocoa solids and cocoa butter. Cocoa liquor is what is referred to as "percent cacao" on food packaging. Cocoa powder is made by removing some of the cocoa butter from the liquor.

Chocolate is a solid food made by combining cocoa liquor with cocoa butter and sugar. The proportion of cocoa liquor in the final product determines how dark the chocolate is. Milk chocolate, typically containing 10%–12% cocoa liquor, is made with the addition of condensed or powdered milk to the chocolate mixture and is the chocolate consumed most in the United States. Semisweet or bittersweet chocolate is often referred to as dark chocolate and must contain no less than 35% by weight of cocoa liquor.

Raw unprocessed cocoa is one of the richest antioxidant foods in the world. Studies indicate that cocoa has an effect on carbon dioxide levels that affect blood vessels and improve blood flow. This has positive implications, for example, on reducing the risk of stroke.

---

[493] Wood, G.A.R.; Lass, R.A. (2001). *Cocoa* (4th ed.). Oxford: Blackwell Science.

Cocoa is a rich source of polyphenols, mainly flavanols, which have been recognized for having positive effects on vascular disease, cancer, diabetes, inflammation, oxidative stress, and blood pressure[494]. Because flavanols have the capacity to cross the

> *A tablespoon of cocoa nibs is an excellent mood food; addition, for example, to frozen banana "ice cream" is a tasty dessert.*

blood-brain barrier, enhancing brain blood flow through the increased production of NO, which has been proposed as a mechanism involved in brain health[495]

Any form other than raw typically contains added fat and sugar and is to be avoided.

Overall, research to date suggests that the benefits of moderate cocoa or dark chocolate consumption likely outweigh the risks of obesity and glycemic load.

HERBS AND SPICES

Choosing fruits and vegetables by color is an excellent way to get a variety of nutritional components, as the colors are related to the nutrition, particularly anti-oxidants. The same can be said for taste and flavors; it appears the more intense

---

[494] Shrime, M. G., Bauer, S. R., Mcdonald, A. C., Chowdhury, N. H., Coltart, C. E., & Ding, E. L. (2011). Flavonoid-Rich Cocoa Consumption Affects Multiple Cardiovascular Risk Factors in a Meta-Analysis of Short-Term Studies. *Journal of Nutrition, 141*(11), 1982-1988. doi:10.3945/jn.111.145482.

[495] Nehlig, A. (2012). The neuroprotective effects of cocoa flavanol and its influence on cognitive performance. *British Journal of Clinical Pharmacology Br J Clin Pharmacol.* doi:10.1111/j.1365-2125.2012.04378.x.

the taste and flavor, the higher the concentration of secondary metabolites and phytonutrient content.

Herbs and spices are plants or plant parts that are particularly intense in their taste or flavor. *Herbs* refer to the leafy green or flowering parts of a plant, while *spices* are produced from other parts of the plant, including seeds, berries, and roots.

Therefore, it follows that small quantities of herbs and spices are typically favored by the consumer and yet they are large in nutrient content.

While any of the foods mentioned in this chapter could be termed nutraceutics, or psychotropic nutraceuticals, traditionally in medicine it is herbs and spices administered in small doses like pharmaceutics that have been consider medicinal.

TURMERIC

Turmeric is a spice with perhaps the highest antioxidant and anti-inflammatory properties of any culinary spice – or herb. One active component of turmeric is curcumin (the pigment responsible for the bright yellow color of the spice), which may have natural antidepressant qualities and has been shown to protect neurons from the damaging effects of chronic stress.

The beneficial effects of curcumin in the pathophysiology of major depression are probably related to its anti-inflammatory and antioxidant properties, inhibition of monoamine oxidase[496], and modulation of neurotrophic factors and hippocampal neurogenesis and neuroplasticity[497].

In a randomized controlled trial[498] , a comparable efficacy was obtained after curcumin monotherapy (1000 mg/day) compared to fluoxetine monotherapy. Supplementation of conventional antidepressants with curcumin (1000 mg/ day) has shown to be an effective and safe enhancement[499].

Meta-analysis of data from the six clinical trials[500] revealed a significant reduction in major depressive symptoms following the administration of curcumin in combination with piperdine (see below). These studies all used the 1000 mg/ day and the anti-depressant effect was best after a duration of six weeks.

---

[496] Kulkarni, S. K., Bhutani, M. K., & Bishnoi, M. (2008). Antidepressant activity of curcumin: Involvement of serotonin and dopamine system. *Psychopharmacology, 201*(3), 435-442. doi:10.1007/s00213-008-1300-y.

[497] Liu, D., Wang, Z., Gao, Z., Xie, K., Zhang, Q., Jiang, H., & Pang, Q. (2014). Effects of curcumin on learning and memory deficits, BDNF, and ERK protein expression in rats exposed to chronic unpredictable stress. *Behavioural Brain Research, 271,* 116-121. doi:10.1016/ j.bbr.2014.05.068.

[498] Sanmukhani, J., Satodia, V., Trivedi, J., Patel, T., Tiwari, D., Panchal, B., . . . Tripathi, C. B. (2013). Efficacy and Safety of Curcumin in Major Depressive Disorder: A Randomized Controlled Trial. *Phytother. Res. Phytotherapy Research, 28*(4), 579-585. doi:10.1002/ptr.5025.

[499] Yu, J., Pei, L., Zhang, Y., Wen, Z., & Yang, J. (2015). Chronic Supplementation of Curcumin Enhances the Efficacy of Antidepressants in Major Depressive Disorder. *Journal of Clinical Psychopharmacology, 1.* doi:10.1097/jcp.0000000000000352.

[500] Al-Karawi, D., Mamoori, D. A., & Tayyar, Y. (2015). The Role of Curcumin Administration in Patients with Major Depressive Disorder: Mini Meta-Analysis of Clinical Trials. *Phytother. Res. Phytotherapy Research, 30*(2), 175-183. doi:10.1002/ptr.5524.

Turmeric suppresses pain and inflammation similar to non-steroidal anti-inflammatories but without the potential side effects. The health benefits derive, as for Rhodiola and Maca, from "xenohormesis" – a biological principle that explains why environmentally stressed plants produce bioactive compounds that can confer stress resistance and survival benefits to animals that consume them (see Chapter 6).

Turmeric contains about 2% by weight curcumin, so a tablespoon of turmeric (6.8 grams) contains about 136 mg of curcumin. To get 1000 mg/ day curcumin from raw turmeric would then require more than seven tablespoons. Supplements that purport to contain 500 mg curcumin are commercially available.

One tablespoon of turmeric (1000 mg) per day with a pinch or two of ground pepper (see below) is recommended. If you grate the turmeric root yourself, be prepared to wear gloves as the color is so intense you will have yellow finger tips otherwise.

GROUND PEPPERCORNS

Black pepper has an ancient history of being a highly desirable but expensive spice. It has even been used as a currency.

Piperine is a simple and pungent alkaloid found in the seeds of black pepper. Piperine is commonly known as a bioavailability enhancer for a number of nutraceuticals, including antioxidants[501] and anti-inflammatories[502], as well as for its

---

[501] Johnson, J. J., Nihal, M., Siddiqui, I. A., Scarlett, C. O., Bailey, H. H., Mukhtar, H., & Ahmad, N. (2011). Enhancing the bioavailability of resveratrol by combining it with piperine. *Molecular Nutrition & Food Research Mol. Nutr. Food Res., 55*(8), 1169-1176. doi:10.1002/mnfr.201100117.

neuroprotective activity[503]. *The Journal of Food and Chemical Toxicology* reported that the compound piperine in black pepper increases the cognitive function of the brain and helps mood disorder.

Piperine helps the body absorb curcumin and therefore enhances curcumin's antidepressant effect long-term. There may be similar absorption assistance given to selenium, vitamin B12, and beta-carotene.

Piperine has shown multiple mechanisms of action, including inhibition of MAO enzymes, elevation of brain serotonin (5-HT) brain derived neurotropic factor (BDNF) levels, and modulation of HPA axis[504].

Because of its intense taste in small quantities, it is typically used as just a few "pinches" into turmeric recipes.

Typically 2.5 mg/ kg is used so for a 70 kg person that would equal 175 mg; a teaspoon of black pepper weighs about 2000 mg, so this is less than 10% of a teaspoon – otherwise known as a "pinch" or two.

---

[502] Ying, X., Yu, K., Chen, X., Chen, H., Hong, J., Cheng, S., & Peng, L. (2013). Piperine inhibits LPS induced expression of inflammatory mediators in RAW 264.7 cells. *Cellular Immunology, 285*(1-2), 49-54. doi:10.1016/j.cellimm.2013.09.001.

[503] Shrivastava, P., Vaibhav, K., Tabassum, R., Khan, A., Ishrat, T., Khan, M. M., . . . Islam, F. (2013). Anti-apoptotic and Anti-inflammatory effect of Piperine on 6-OHDA induced Parkinson's Rat model. *The Journal of Nutritional Biochemistry, 24*(4), 680-687. doi:10.1016/ j.jnutbio.2012.03.018

[504] Mao, Q.Q., Xian, Y.F., Ip, S.P., and Che, C.T. (2011). Involvement of serotonergic system in the antidepressant-like effect of piperine. Prog. Neuropsychopharmacol. Biol. Psychiatry 35, 1144–1147

SAFFRON

According to ancient Greek mythology, Hermes and his friend Krokos were engaged in horseplay when Hermes accidentally killed Krokos by head injury, with three blood drops from his head falling on the top of a flower, creating three stigmata and naming this plant thereafter Krokos (Crocus)[505]. Thus the ancient and godly identification of this plant.

Saffron is the dried stigma (the top part in the center of a flower which receives the pollen and on which germination takes place) of the blue-purple flower Crocus sativus L., and it has a long history of use as a spice, coloring agent, and medicine. Due to how saffron is grown and harvested, saffron is considered one of the world's most expensive spices (upwards of $11,000 per kg, requiring 450,000 hand-picked stigmas)[506]. Apart from its traditional value as a spice and coloring agent (originally for the Persian carpet industry), saffron has a long history of medicinal use spanning over 2,500 years[507].

This use of saffron in traditional medicine included for cramps, asthma, menstruation disorders, liver disease, and painful dysmenorrhea[508], among many other uses. Evidence from

---

[505] Koulakiotis, N., Pittenauer, E., Halabalaki, M., Skaltsounis, L., Allmaier, G., & Tsarbopoulos, A. (2011). Isolation and Tandem Mass Spectometric Characterization of Selected Crocus sativus L. (Saffron) Bioactive Compounds.*Planta Med Planta Medica, 77*(12). doi:10.1055/s-0031-1282560.

[506] Gohari, A., Saeidnia, S., & Mahmoodabadi, M. (2013). An overview on saffron, phytochemicals, and medicinal properties. *Pharmacognosy Reviews Phcog Rev,7*(1), 61. doi:10.4103/0973-7847.112850.

[507] Srivastava, R., Ahmed, H., Dixit, R., D., & Saraf, S. (2010). Crocus sativus L.: A comprehensive review. *Pharmacognosy Reviews, 4*(8), 200. doi:10.4103/0973-7847.70919.

[508] Kianbakht, S., & Ghazavi, A. (2011). Immunomodulatory Effects of Saffron: A Randomized Double-Blind Placebo-Controlled Clinical Tri-

recent *in vitro* and *in vivo* research indicates that saffron has potential anti-carcinogenic, anti-mutagenic, antioxidant, and memory-enhancing properties[509] [510].

Neurodegenerative disorders

Administration of saffron 30 mg/day (15 mg twice daily) was found to be as effective as a leading medication for mild to moderate Alzheimer's disease (donepezil) in a placebo-controlled double-blind study in subjects 55 years and older[511], but with a better side-effect profile. Although there are a growing number of non-human animal studies and theories why saffron could be neuroprotective for Alzheimer 's disease and other neurodegenerative conditions, clinical studies are too few to make even tentative conclusions to date.

---

al. *Phytother. Res. Phytotherapy Research, 25*(12), 1801-1805. doi:10.1002/ptr.3484.

[509] Abdullaev, F., & Espinosa-Aguirre, J. (2004). Biomedical properties of saffron and its potential use in cancer therapy and chemoprevention trials. *Cancer Detection and Prevention, 28*(6), 426-432. doi:10.1016/j.cdp.2004.09.002.

[510] Bathaie, S. Z., & Mousavi, S. Z. (2010). New Applications and Mechanisms of Action of Saffron and its Important Ingredients. *Critical Reviews in Food Science and Nutrition, 50*(8), 761-786. doi:10.1080/10408390902773003.

[511] Akhondzadeh, S., Sabet, M. S., Harirchian, M. H., Togha, M., Cheraghmakani, H., Razeghi, S., . . . Moradi, A. (2010). ORIGINAL ARTI-CLE: Saffron in the treatment of patients with mild to moderate Alz-heimer's disease: A 16-week, randomized and placebo-controlled trial. *Journal of Clinical Pharmacy and Therapeutics, 35*(5), 581-588. doi:10.1111/j.1365-2710.2009.01133.x.

Mood disorders

In two randomized, double-blind, placebo-controlled trials, saffron was effective for the treatment of mild to moderate depression[512][513].

A systematic review of randomized control trials examining the effectiveness of saffron in mood disorders revealed a statistically significant effect on improved mood on subjects clinically diagnosed with depression[514]; the dosing was typically 30 mg/ day.

In clinical studies, the use of saffron extract at doses of 20–30 mg/day twice daily for the treatment of mild to moderate depression has been compared with currently marketed antidepressants such as fluoxetine[515] (20 mg/day twice daily)

---

[512] Akhondzadeh, S., Tahmacebi-Pour, N., Noorbala, A., Amini, H., Fal-lah-Pour, H., Jamshidi, A., & Khani, M. (2005). Crocus sativus L. in the treatment of mild to moderate depression: A double-blind, randomized and placebo-controlled trial. *Phytother. Res. Phytotherapy Research, 19*(2), 148-151. doi:10.1002/ptr.1647.

[513] Moshiri, E., Basti, A. A., Noorbala, A., Jamshidi, A., Abbasi, S. H., & Akhondzadeh, S. (2006). Crocus sativus L. (petal) in the treatment of mild-to-moderate depression: A double-blind, randomized and placebo-controlled trial. *Phytomedicine, 13*(9-10), 607-611. doi:10.1016/j.phymed.2006.08.006.

[514] Hausenblas, H. A., Heekin, K., Mutchie, H. L., & Anton, S. (2015). A systematic review of randomized controlled trials examining the effec-tiveness of saffron (Crocus sativus L.) on psychological and behavioral outcomes. *Journal of Integrative Medicine, 13*(4), 231-240. doi:10.1016/s2095-4964(15)60176-5.

[515] Noorbala, A., Akhondzadeh, S., Tahmacebi-Pour, N., & Jamshidi, A. (2005). Hydro-alcoholic extract of Crocus sativus L. versus fluoxetine in the treatment of mild to moderate depression: A double-blind, random-ized pilot trial. *Journal of Ethnopharmacology, 97*(2), 281-284. doi:10.1016/j.jep.2004.11.004.

and imipramine[516] (100 mg/day three times daily). So these comparative evaluations revealed that saffron was equally as effective as chemically synthesized marketed pharmaceutics in mild or moderate depression without causing the typical side effects of the artificial preparations.

Saffron may act in a manner similar to antidepressants to improve mood by inhibiting serotonin reuptake[517] or there could be multiple pathways involving, for example, its antioxidant, anti-inflammatory properties.

Saffron contains in excess of 150 volatile and aroma-yielding compounds and many non-volatile active components, many of which are carotenoids[518] . Safranal is the compound primarily responsible for saffron's aroma. Safranal has shown to have anti-convulsant and anxiolytic effects[519] as well as antidepressant properties[520].

---

[516] Akhondzadeh, S., Fallah-Pour, H., Afkham, K., Jamshidi, A., & Kha-lighi-Cigaroudi, F. (2004). Comparison of Crocus sativus L. and imipramine in the treatment of mild to moderate depression: A pilot double-blind randomized trial [ISRCTN45683816]. *BMC Complementary and Alternative Medicine BMC Complement Altern Med, 4*(1). doi:10.1186/1472-6882-4-12.

[517] Hausenblas, H. A., Saha, D., Dubyak, P. J., & Anton, S. D. (2013). Saffron (Crocus sativus L.) and major depressive disorder: A meta-analysis of randomized clinical trials. *Journal of Integrative Medicine, 11*(6), 377-383. doi:10.3736/jintegrmed2013056.

[518] Sampathu, S. R., Shivashankar, S., Lewis, Y. S., & Wood, A. B. (1984). Saffron (Crocus Sativus Linn.) — Cultivation, processing, chemistry and standardization.*C R C Critical Reviews in Food Science and Nutrition, 20*(2), 123-157. doi:10.1080/10408398409527386

[519] Hosseinzadeh, H., & Talebzadeh, F. (2005). Anticonvulsant evaluation of safranal and crocin from Crocus sativus in mice. *Fitoterapia, 76*(7-8), 722-724. doi:10.1016/j.fitote.2005.07.008.

[520] Hosseinzadeh, H., Karimi, G., & Niapoor, M. (2004). Antidepressant Effect Of Crocus Sativus L. Stigma Extracts And Their Constituents,

Premenstrual Syndrome (PMS)

One randomized controlled trial examined the effects of saffron supplementation on premenstrual syndrome[521]. It was found that women with regular menstrual cycles experiencing premenstrual syndrome who took 30 mg/day of saffron supplementation for eight weeks reported relief in premenstrual symptoms and depression levels compared to placebo. Remarkably, just the aroma alone – without otherwise any oral intake of saffron was found effective in relief of PMS symptoms in another placebo-controlled double-blind study[522], indicating effectiveness at very small doses.

HIBISCUS FLOWERS

Flowers of Hibiscus (rosa-sinensis Linn) popularly known as "China-rose flowers" contain significant flavonoids (such as anthocyanin and quercetin) known to have antidepressant activity[523].

Crocin And Safranal, In Mice. *Acta Hortic. Acta Horticulturae,* (650), 435-445. doi:10.17660/actahortic.2004.650.54.

[521] Agha-Hosseini, M., Kashani, L., Aleyaseen, A., Ghoreishi, A., Rahmanpour, H., Zarrinara, A., & Akhondzadeh, S. (2008). Crocus sativus L. (saffron) in the treatment of premenstrual syndrome: A double-blind, randomised and placebo-controlled trial. *BJOG: Int J O & G BJOG: An International Journal of Obstetrics and Gynaecology, 115*(4), 515-519. doi:10.1111/j.1471-0528.2007.01652.x.

[522] Fukui, H., Toyoshima, K., & Komaki, R. (2011). Psychological and neuroendocrinological effects of odor of saffron (Crocus sativus).*Phytomedicine, 18*(8-9), 726-730. doi:10.1016/ j.phymed. 2010.11.013.

[523] Butterweck, V., Jürgenliemk, G., Nahrstedt, A., & Winterhoff, H. (2000). Flavonoids from Hypericum perforatum Show Antidepressant Activity in the Forced Swimming Test. *Planta Medica, 66*(1), 3-6. doi:10.1055/s-2000-11119.

The antidepressant effect may be from its antioxidant activity[524]; there are few controlled studies on human populations. Hibiscus has been used in Hawaiian cultures to treat postpartum depression[525].

Another herbal tea, made from the sepals of Hibiscus flowers are beautiful, showy red flowers that are harvested and dried like most teas. This plant contains bioflavonoids, which are believed to help prevent an increase in LDL cholesterol, and to lower blood pressure[526]. The research is quite clear on these effects. It may work by boosting nitric oxide production, generally an advantage for cardiovascular activities.

Again, why bother to make tea with this food and limit the nutrient availability when you can eat it! I use a heaping tablespoon in my morning smoothie. I also like to blend it with green tea and ice, then strain it into water bottles as a drink during exercise.

ROOIBOS

Rooibos (Aspalathus linearis) is a bush native to the Cedarberg Mountains in the Western Cape region of South Africa where it is extensively cultivated for its commercial use as an herbal tea. After harvesting, the needle-like leaves and stems can be either

---

[524] Vanzella, C., Bianchetti, P., Sbaraini, S., Vanzin, S. I., Melecchi, M. I., Caramão, E. B., & Siqueira, I. R. (2012). Antidepressant-like effects of methanol extract of Hibiscus tiliaceus flowers in mice. *BMC Complementary and Alternative Medicine, 12*(1). doi:10.1186/1472-6882-12-41.

[525] Kobayashi, J. (1976). Early Hawaiian Uses of Medicinal Plants in Pregnancy and Childbirth. *Journal of Tropical Pediatrics, 22*(6), 260-262. doi:10.1093/tropej/22.6.260.

[526] Siddiqui, A., Wani, S., Rajesh, R., & Alagarsamy, V. (2006). Phytochemical and pharmacological investigation of flowers of hibiscus rosas-inensis linn. *Indian Journal of Pharmaceutical Sciences Indian J Pharm Sci, 68*(1), 127. doi:10.4103/0250-474x.22986.

fermented prior to drying or dried immediately. The unfermented product remains green in color and is referred to as green rooibos. During fermentation, the color changes from green to red with oxidation of the constituent polyphenols, so the final product is often referred to as "red tea" or "red bush tea." The non-oxidized green version, let's call it "green herbal tea," would be superior in antioxidants.

Rooibos possesses antimutagenic, anticarcinogenic, anti-inflammatory and antiviral activity[527], as does unfermented green herbal tea.

Rooibos is especially rich in the super-antioxidant compound quercetin. Rooibos is a source of two comparatively rare antioxidants, aspalathin and nothofagin. Aspalathin helps to modify hormones in the body and reduces the output of adrenal hormones, thus reducing stress and helping to inhibit metabolic disorders. The antioxidant nothofagin demonstrates significant anti-inflammatory activity and neuroprotective functions[528].

As this is a tea, why not buy teabags, add hot water and drink it? Well that's fine, but much more expensive than bulk purchase. While the process of preparing, serving, and sipping tea can be an art, we are here interested in the nutrient value – and efficiency of preparation. Steeping in hot water extracts only a portion of the water-soluble components (such as polyphenols) of the plant, i.e., that which enters into solution if

[527] Joubert, E., Gelderblom, W., Louw, A., & Beer, D. D. (2008). South African herbal teas: Aspalathus linearis, Cyclopia spp. and Athrixia phyli-coides - A review. *Journal of Ethnopharmacology, 119*(3), 376-412. doi:10.1016/j.jep.2008.06.014.
[528] Mckay, D. L., & Blumberg, J. B. (2006). A review of the bioactivity of south African herbal teas: Rooibos (Aspalathus linearis) and honey-bush (Cyclopia intermedia). *Phytother. Res. Phytotherapy Research, 21*(1), 1-16. doi:10.1002/ptr.1992.

the fibrous cell walls are sufficiently disrupted by the heating process – the rest is discarded in the tea bag.

But as a food, the entire leaf can be eaten and all nutrients consumed. A dose suggested from literature studies is one teaspoon.

RHODIOLA

A systematic review of numerous randomized placebo-controlled studies of Rhodiola rosea showed beneficial effects on physical performance, mental performance, and in mild to moderate depression[529]. For example, one Swedish phase II randomized placebo-controlled study over a six-week clinical trial concluded[530]:

> *"R. rosea possesses a clear and significant anti-depressive activity in patients suffering from mild to moderate depression. When administered in a dosage of two tablets, each containing 170 mg of extract, daily over a 6-week period, statistical significant reduction in the overall symptom level of depression as well as in specific symptoms of depression, such as insomnia, emotional instability and somatization, could be demonstrated. In higher doses, four tablets per day over a 6-week period, an additional positive effect could be*

---

[529] Hung, S. K., Perry, R., & Ernst, E. (2011). The effectiveness and efficacy of Rhodiola rosea L.: A systematic review of randomized clinical trials. *Phytomedicine, 18*(4), 235-244. doi:10.1016/ j.phymed. 2010.08.014.

[530] Darbinyan, V., Aslanyan, G., Amroyan, E., Gabrielyan, E., Malmström, C., & Panossian, A. (2007). Clinical trial of Rhodiola rosea L. extract SHR-5 in the treatment of mild to moderate depression. *Nordic Journal of Psychiatry, 61*(5), 343-348. doi:10.1080/08039480701643290.

shown. No side-effects resulting from treatment could be detected in any group of the groups".

Therefore, doses of about 300 – 600 mg were effective in that study.

The mechanism of action may be inhibition of monoamine re-uptake (such as serotonin, dopamine and noradrenaline), enhanced binding and sensitization of serotonin receptors, monoamine oxidase inhibition, and neuro-endocrine modulation[531]. Rhodiola is apparently adaptogenic, meaning that it does its good deeds without disturbing normal biologic functions.

I'm not sure if it is an herb (plant leaf, stem, or flower used for flavoring or medicinal use) or a spice (same as herb but a root). The aerial portion (above ground plant) is used as a food. However, various alternative names for the plant include "root," such as the "red root" and the powder is a deep red so I assume that the medicinal part is primarily a root and therefore technically a spice.

Rhodiola Rosea 3% Salidroside Powder (100 grams) costs about $18[532]. I use a little less than one eighth of a teaspoon, about 300 mg (a cost of about ten cents). I'm unsure of where this was harvested although it can grow on cold rocky slopes in the USA; it has been suggested to aid those living in very cold

---

[531] Kumar, V. (2006). Potential medicinal plants for CNS disorders: An overview.*Phytother. Res. Phytotherapy Research, 20*(12), 1023-1035. doi:10.1002/ptr.1970

[532] My source for this is from Bulk Supplements (www.bulksupplements.com) – I order from Amazon and guided in my selection in part by happy consumers who have tried it and like it on some basis.

stressful environments where it grows, such as Siberia and Scandinavia. It has a shelf life of three or more years.

MACA root

Maca has been cultivated and grown high in the Andean Mountains of Peru for thousands of years.

Like Rhodiola, it flourishes in extreme environments of freezing cold winds, strong sunlight, and high elevation (over 10,000 feet). There does appear to be a correlation between plants that survive in stressful circumstances and the adaptogenic effects that such plants have on the human body and mind.

The root of the maca plant has been used for centuries as a nutritive substance that raises the body's state of resistance to disease by increasing immunity to stress while remaining nontoxic to the recipient.

The shelf life is an amazing seven years. Maca is powerfully abundant in amino acids, phytonutrients, healthy fatty acids, vitamins, and minerals. This superfood allegedly has the ability to increase energy and stamina, working directly on the hypothalamus and pituitary glands.

Once again, there are some indications of positive effect on mood[533].

About two tablespoons of maca powered root was used in the above studies. A good source of maca is the "premium"

---

[533] Rubio, J., Caldas, M., Dávila, S., Gasco, M., & Gonzales, G. F. (2006). Effect of three different cultivars of Lepidium meyenii (Maca) on learning and depression in ovariectomized mice. *BMC Complementary and Alternative Medicine BMC Complement Altern Med, 6*(1). doi:10.1186/1472-6882-6-23.

combination of Peruvian sources from "The Maca Team" available on the internet.

ASHWAGANDHA ROOTS (WITHANIA SOMNIFERA)

The root of Withania somnifera is used extensively in Ayurveda, the classical Indian system of medicine, and is categorized as a rasayana, an herbal remedy used to promote physical and mental health[534].

There are many claims concerning the health benefits of Ashwagandha root and most all of them concern reduction of adrenal stress (anxiety) and reduction of inflammation; there are many peer reviewed studies, including systematic review summaries that are rather convincing. Positive influences on neurodegenerative diseases such as cognitive decline and dementias have been suggested[535].

There are plenty of herbs and spices with demonstrated powerful psychotropic nutraceutical effects.

It is likely helpful to ingest this substance after exercise, particularly endurance workouts or heavy lifting (supposedly it helps to stimulate muscle recovery).

Also this Ayurvedic has been used to help treat insomnia.

---

[534] Bhattacharya, S., Bhattacharya, A., Sairam, K., & Ghosal, S. (2000). Anxiolytic-antidepressant activity of Withania somnifera glycowithanolides: An experimental study. *Phytomedicine, 7*(6), 463-469. doi:10.1016/ s0944-7113(00)80030-6.

[535] Manchanda, S., Mishra, R., Singh, R., Kaur, T., & Kaur, G. (2016). Aqueous Leaf Extract of Withania somnifera as a Potential Neuroprotective Agent in Sleep-deprived Rats: A Mechanistic Study. *Molecular Neurobiology Mol Neurobiol*. doi:10.1007/s12035-016-9883-5.

The amount suggested by the literature studies is one-half teaspoon, about 1600 mg.

SUPPLEMENTS

While this book recommends a whole-food varied-plant dietary patterns, there are a few supplements that may be important to some individuals who cannot get certain nutrients in their food.

VITAMIN B_{12}

An argument often given against adoption of a whole-food varied-plant diet is that it doesn't provide vitamin B_{12}. How can it be that primates could exist for most of the past 85 million years eating only fruits and vegetables if they could not get this essential nutrient?

Plants cannot produce vitamin B_{12}, but neither can animals, or fungi for that matter. Only certain bacteria (plus *archaea,* now classified as a prokaryote distinct from bacteria) can produce it; we can't even synthesize this complex molecule in the laboratory. The soil bacteria called *Rhizobia* that fixes nitrogen after being taken in by plant root nodules make it[536]. Herbivores get their B_{12} from eating the plants that contain those bacteria. Carnivores get their B_{12} by consuming herbivores. Once in the animal gut, the bacteria can apparently proliferate and the nutrient is manufactured in the large intestine.

However, unfortunately, it isn't absorbed there as such absorption would have to occur in the small intestine.

---

[536] Herbert, V. (1988). Vitamin B-12: Plant sources, requirements, and assay. *The American Journal of Clinical Nutrition, 48*(3), 852-858.

Therefore, the abundant supply of this essential nutrient appears in animal feces, including that of insects. This makes its way onto the external surfaces of plants and into springs and streams carrying animal excrement.

In our more hygienic world of Western society, we take special measure to wash plant parts, removing the B_{12}. Similarly our water supplies are treated to remove bacteria. Pesticides, herbicides, and other chemicals used to treat our modern mass produced produce reduce the amount of this bacteria that can grow in our soils. So the fact that whole-food varied-plant diets are devoid of B_{12} is not based on genetic mutations or a need to eat animal products but on good hygiene and bad farming practices.

A supplement for B_{12} is recommended for individuals on whole-food varied-plant diets.

VITAMIN D

The fourth vitamin to be discovered, vitamin D, is technically not a vitamin as one's body can produce it – it just requires sunlight. No one is suggesting that sunlight is a vitamin per se. Only a relatively short span of radiation from the sun is involved, the so-called UVB of the ultraviolet spectrum. The intensity of UVB available depends on the weather, season, location on earth, and time of day; in the United States it maximizes between 10 am and 4 pm in April through October.

With moderate direct exposure to the summer sun (say 5 - 30 minutes twice a week), the body will make 10,000 to 20,000 IU of vitamin D. Sunscreen can effectively block UVB absorption; for an individual with frequent sun exposure (greater than twice per week), it might be prudent to use sunscreen after the first 10 – 15 minutes of sun exposure to avoid skin cancer but allow vitamin D production. As our bodies can store vitamin D, it is thought that sufficient exposure during spring, summer, and early fall should be sufficient to provide needed vitamin D during the winter months.

So this is another relatively recent modification in our evolution – to stay indoors a lot more than our ancestors, decreasing our vitamin D production. The National Academies Institute of Medicine has no guidelines for vitamin D through sun exposure; it does have an RDA, but it is based on food intake.

The reaction of cholesterol (in the form of 7-dehydrocholesterol) in the skin with sunlight actually produces several fat-soluble related compounds, the most important being cholecalciferol, vitamin D_3, and ergocalciferol, vitamin D_2. The term "vitamin D" includes both of these compounds.

Very few foods in nature contain vitamin D, although some food products have vitamin D as an additive. To manufacture vitamin D industrially, 7-dehydrocholesterol, a substance typically obtained from fish liver[537] or lanolin extracted from shorn sheep wool, is exposed to UVB light, producing vitamin D_3. Vitamin D cannot be manufactured directly; it requires the photochemical process.

Little is known about which species or groups of phytoplanktonic algae are capable of vitamin D synthesis, since only natural mixtures of algae and a few defined species have been analyzed. Apparently reindeer lichen contains vitamin D_2 and vitamin D_3[538]; the food source for the lichen is unclear.

---

[537] Takeuchi A, Okano T, Sayamoto M, Sawamura S, Kobayashi T, Motosugi M, Yamakawa T; Okano; Sayamoto; Sawamura; Kobayashi; Motosugi; Yamakawa (1986). "Tissue distribution of 7-dehydrocholesterol, vitamin D3 and 25-hydroxyvitamin D3 in several species of fishes". *Journal of nutritional science and vitaminology.* **32** (1): 13–22.

[538] Bjorn, L. and T. Wang (2000). "Vitamin D in an ecological context". Int J Circumpolar Health **59** (1): 26 – 32.

Vitamin D precursors are synthesized by some higher plants, apparently acting as a growth substance[539]. Provitamin D_2 is synthesized by many fungi, and this fact may explain some traits of plant-fungal symbiosis.

Vitamin D precursors can be industrially manufactured but is rather expensive, utilizing molybdenum catalysis[540].

To become biologically active, vitamin D has to undergo two transformative reactions, one in the liver, then another in the kidney.

Vitamin D deficiency to the extent of causing rickets or osteomalacia is rare in the developed world but what we might call vitamin D insufficiency, a lower than ideal biologically active form of vitamin D, appears to be quite common, particularly in the elderly.

Vitamin D toxicity is also rare. There is a feedback loop associated with vitamin D production in the skin that lowers its production as adequate amounts are reached. This natural regulatory mechanism doesn't apply to supplementation but for daily supplemental intake of 2,000 IU (about 50 micrograms) per day, there is very little risk of toxicity.[541]

---

[539] Baur, A. C., Brandsch, C., König, B., Hirche, F., & Stangl, G. I. (2016). Plant Oils as Potential Sources of Vitamin D. *Frontiers in Nutrition, 3*. doi:10.3389/fnut.2016.00029.
[540] Rahman, F. U., & Tan, T. W. (2011). Synthesis of 7-dehydrocholesterol through hexacarbonyl molybdenum catalyzed elimination reaction. *Bulletin of the Chemical Society of Ethiopia Bull. Chem. Soc. Eth., 25*(2). doi:10.4314/bcse.v25i2.65899.
[541] Ross, A. C., Manson, J. E., Abrams, S. A., Aloia, J. F., Brannon, P. M., Clinton, S. K., . . . Shapses, S. A. (2011). The 2011 Dietary Reference Intakes for Calcium and Vitamin D: What Dietetics Practitioners Need to Know. This article is a summary of the Institute of Medicine report entitled Dietary Reference Intakes for Calcium and Vitamin D (available at

As vitamin D is fat soluble, it requires the presence of fat for absorption; some supplements encapsulate cholecalciferol, vitamin D_3, with fat; otherwise often it is recommended to take with a meal containing some fat.

We have learned relatively recently that vitamin D has a much larger effect on the body than just calcium absorption; for example, it has to do with modulation of cell growth, neuromuscular and immune function, and reduction of inflammation[542]. And mood states.

Vitamin D and psychiatric disorders

Vitamin D acts on receptors in a variety of regions in the brain such as the prefrontal cortex, hippocampus, cingulate gyrus, thalamus, hypothalamus, and substantia nigra and as such can influence neurochemistry[543], cognition, emotion, and behavior. Vitamin D deficiency in early life affects neuronal

---

http://www.iom.edu/Reports/2010/Dietary-Reference-Intakes-for-Calcium-and-Vitamin-D.aspx) for dietetics practitioners; a similar summary for clinicians has also been published (Ross AC, Manson JE, Abrams SA, Aloia JF, Brannon PM, Clinton SK, Durazo-Arvizu RA, Gallagher JC, Gallo RL, Jones G, Kovacs CS, Mayne ST, Rosen CJ, Shapses SA. The 2011 report on Dietary Reference Intakes for calcium and vitamin D from the Institute of Medicine: What clinicians need to know. J Clin Endocrinol Metab. 2011;96:53-58).*Journal of the American Dietetic Association, 111*(4), 524-527. doi:10.1016/j.jada.2011.01.004.

[542] DRI – Dietary Reference Intakes – Calcium and Vitamin D20122 DRI – Dietary Reference Intakes – Calcium and Vitamin D . Institute of Medicine of the National Academies, , ISBN: 13-978-0-309-16394-1. (2012). *Nutrition & Food Science, 42*(2), 131-131. doi:10.1108/nfs.2012.42.2.131.2.

[543] Yue, W., Xiang, L., Zhang, Y., Ji, Y., & Li, X. (2014). Association of Serum 25-Hydroxyvitamin D with Symptoms of Depression After 6 Months in Stroke Patients. *Neurochem Res Neurochemical Research, 39*(11), 2218-2224. doi:10.1007/s11064-014-1423-y.

differentiation, brain structure and function, and appears to have some influence on disorders with a developmental basis, such as autistic spectrum disorder ,schizophrenia ontogeny and brain structure and function[544].

The initial suggestion that vitamin D may be linked to clinical depression was based on the relation between low vitamin D and high prevalence of seasonal affective disorder (now considered to be a depressive disorder with seasonal pattern[545]) in winter at high latitudes[546]. One treatment modality for clinical depression with seasonal pattern is light therapy, although no ultra-violet light is used. Vitamin D insufficiency is not considered to be directly causative for clinical depression with seasonal pattern.

However, vitamin D concentrations have been shown to be low in many patients suffering from mood disorders and have been associated with poor cognitive function[547] [548]. For example,

---

[544] Eyles, D. W., Burne, T. H., & Mcgrath, J. J. (2013). Vitamin D, effects on brain development, adult brain function and the links between low levels of vitamin D and neuropsychiatric disease. *Frontiers in Neuroendocrinology, 34*(1), 47-64. doi:10.1016/j.yfrne.2012.07.001.

[545] Gabbard, Glen O. *Treatment of Psychiatric Disorders.* **2** (3rd ed.). Washington, DC: American Psychiatric Publishing. p. 1296.

[546] Stumpf WE, Privette TH: Light, vitamin D and psychiatry. Role of 1,25 dihydroxyvitamin D3 (soltriol) in etiology and therapy of seasonal affective disorder and other mental processes. Psychopharmacology (Berl) 1989, 97:285–294.

[547] Wilkins, C. H., Sheline, Y. I., Roe, C. M., Birge, S. J., & Morris, J. C. (2006). Vitamin D Deficiency Is Associated With Low Mood and Worse Cognitive Performance in Older Adults. *The American Journal of Geriatric Psychiatry, 14*(12), 1032-1040. doi:10.1097/ 01.jgp.0000240986. 74642.7c.

[548] Przybelski, R. J., & Binkley, N. C. (2007). Is vitamin D important for preserving cognition? A positive correlation of serum 25-hydroxyvitamin D concentration with cognitive function. *Archives of Biochemistry and Biophysics, 460*(2), 202-205. doi:10.1016/j.abb.2006.12.018.

data from the third National Health and Nutrition Examination Survey were used to assess association between serum vitamin D and depression in 7,970 residents of the United States[549]. In that study, the likelihood of having depression in persons with vitamin D insufficiency was found to be significantly higher compared to those with vitamin D sufficiency.

One thorough systematic review and meta-analysis of observational studies and randomized controlled trials was conducted and found that vitamin D insufficiency was strongly associated with clinical depression[550]. Another systematic review and meta-analysis showed a statistically significant improvement in depression with Vitamin D supplements[551].

Use of vitamin D as adjunctive therapy, i.e. together with an antidepressant medication in patients with vitamin D insufficiency has shown to be superior to an antidepressant alone[552].

---

[549] Ganji, V., Milone, C., Cody, M. M., Mccarty, F., & Wang, Y. T. (2010). Serum vitamin D concentrations are related to depression in young adult US population: The Third National Health and Nutrition Examination Survey. *Int Arch Med International Archives of Medicine, 3*(1), 29. doi:10.1186/1755-7682-3-29.

[550] Anglin, R. E., Samaan, Z., Walter, S. D., & Mcdonald, S. D. (2013). Vitamin D deficiency and depression in adults: Systematic review and meta-analysis. *The British Journal of Psychiatry, 202*(2), 100-107. doi:10.1192/bjp.bp.111.106666.

[551] Spedding, S. (2014). Vitamin D and Depression: A Systematic Review and Meta-Analysis Comparing Studies with and without Biological Flaws. *Nutrients, 6*(4), 1501-1518. doi:10.3390/nu6041501.

[552] Khoraminya, N., Tehrani-Doost, M., Jazayeri, S., Hosseini, A., & Djazayery, A. (2012). Therapeutic effects of vitamin D as adjunctive therapy to fluoxetine in patients with major depressive disorder. *Australian & New Zealand Journal of Psychiatry, 47*(3), 271-275. doi:10.1177/0004867412465022.

This is another situation where recent changes in human lifestyle – here being indoors more than outdoors - can lead to a nutrient deficiency. Because it is so common to have a vitamin D insufficiency and the health consequences, specifically mood disorders, I recommend more time in the outdoors, including some limited time (say 10 minutes a day) with face and arms exposure without sunscreen.

If you do not spend regular time in the sun, I do recommend a vitamin D_3 supplement (2000 IU) to be taken before, during, or directly after a meal. I think it wise to take these supplements during the winter months in any case.

Should you question whether or not you may be clinically depressed, professional assessment certainly is recommended. Initial workup may include serum vitamin D levels (usually 25(OH)D is measured but various labs use different techniques resulting in varying "normal" level ranges).

A strict ethical vegan, however, faces a dilemma as the sources of vitamin D_3 supplementation (and all "fortified products such as almond milk and tofu) are animal-based. Some literature supports vitamin D_2 intake as sufficient, but good studies are too scarce to suggest this as the sole source for supplementation; vitamin D_2 can be obtained from certain mushrooms set out in the sun for 10 minutes or so prior to consumption and there are supplements available from this source.

Lichen sources of Vitamin D may hold promise but the food source for the lichen is unclear – it may involve animal break-down products. Future synthetic Vitamin D is likely on the horizon.

It would appear that lifestyle emphasis on "fun in the sun" is best for all, but perhaps particularly for vegans.

OMEGA-3 SUPPLEMENTS

For reasons detailed in this book multiple times, omega-3 intake is critical. The best source is flaxseed. Flaxseed can be bought in bulk form and is inexpensive; after crushing, they can be added to most foods. It is available in crushed form in packets of two tablespoons each, good for the daily requirement.

However, real daily life happens occasionally devoid of your daily dose for one of a myriad of reasons; in this case, rather than just pass on the flaxseeds for the day (or extended periods of time), take a supplement. Two grams per day in capsule form costs about $0.30[553].

IODINE

Iodine, an essential nutrient, is an intrinsic component of the thyroid hormone regulating metabolism at all ages and critical for fetal, infant, and child development, including neurodevelopment[554]. Iodine deficiency is the leading cause of preventable intellectual developmental disability in the world. If iodine intake is chronically too low or too high, prevalence of hypothyroidism or hyperthyroidism may be elevated[555].

The daily Dietary Reference Intake (DRI) recommended by the United States Institute of Medicine is between 110 and

---

[553] For example, Deva Organic Vegan Vitamins Flax Seed Oil.

[554] Delange, F. (2007). Iodine requirements during pregnancy, lactation and the neonatal period and indicators of optimal iodine nutrition. *Public Health Nutrition, 10*(12A). doi:10.1017/s1368980007360941.

[555] Zimmermann, M. B., & Boelaert, K. (2015). Iodine deficiency and thyroid disorders. *The Lancet Diabetes & Endocrinology, 3*(4), 286-295. doi:10.1016/s2213-8587(14)70225-6.

130 µg for infants up to 12 months, 90 µg for children up to eight years, 130 µg for children up to 13 years, 150 µg for adults, 220 µg for pregnant women and 290 µg for lactating mothers[556]. The Tolerable Upper Intake Level for adults is 1,100 µg /day (1.1 mg/day).

Hypothyroidism results in symptoms that appear similar to clinical depression, such as low mood, low energy levels, weight gain, forgetfulness, and personality changes; it can also lead to elevated cholesterol levels.

Hyperthyroidism mimics mania and anxiety disorders, with increased activity and weight loss, difficulty sleeping, and irritability.

Reduction in the prevalence of iodine deficiency worldwide has been achieved through the fortification of sodium chloride ("table salt"; sea salt and salted processed foods are not fortified with iodine), but salting foods leads to increase in blood pressure, the major risk factor for death worldwide. Therefore, if we are not eating salted food or fish, as recommended in our whole-food varied-plant diet, are we getting enough iodine?

In fact, making the dietary iodine sufficiency even more challenging, soy, flaxseed, spinach, sweet potatoes, pears, peaches, raw cruciferous vegetables (broccoli, Brussels sprouts, cauliflower and cabbage), and other fruits and vegetables disrupt the production of thyroid hormones by interfering with

---

[556] United States National Research Council (2000). *Dietary Reference Intakes for Vitamin A, Vitamin K, Arsenic, Boron, Chromium, Copper, Iodine, Iron, Manganese, Molybdenum, Nickel, Silicon, Vanadium, and Zinc.* National Academies Press. pp. 258–259.

iodine uptake in the thyroid gland[557], acting as so-called *goitrogens*.

There are fruits and vegetables that may contain significant levels of iodine, but this is highly dependent on the soil in which the plant was grown. Organic farming tends to yield higher amounts of iodine because there is a greater tendency for proper soil management and crop rotation. Some foods that may contain significant amounts of iodine include:

- Dried seaweed; a quarter ounce serving may contain as much as 4500 μg of iodine – four times the Tolerable Upper Intake Level. Unless you are a regular consumer of high purity seaweed and can adjust the amount to close to the DRI, this should probably not be your dietary source of iodine.

- Potatoes; the skin of a medium size common potato can harbor as much as 60 μg of iodine, so three potatoes could provide adequate daily intake. However, again, it depends on the soil and farming methods as well as the accompanying dietary goitrogens.

- Cranberries; can be rich in iodine with the same provisos as those listed for potatoes.

There are limited data on the dietary iodine intake of vegetarians and vegans in the United States; however, the iodine content of a Swedish vegan diet was found to be 39 μg iodine per 1000 kcal compared to a mixed diet of 156 μg[558] per

---

[557] Vanderpas J (2006). "Nutritional epidemiology and thyroid hormone metabolism". *Annu. Rev. Nutr.* 26: 293–322. doi:10.1146/ annurev.nutr.26.010506.103810.

[558] AbdullaM, Andersson I, Asp NG, Berthelsen K, Birkhed D, Dencker I, Johansson CG, Ja¨ gerstad M, Kolar K, Nair BM, Nilsson-Ehle P, Norde´n

1000 kcal. This was similar to the iodine content of German vegan diets[559].

The first report of iodine nutrition and thyroid function in vegans in the United States stated that Americans are at risk for low iodine intake, and this was for vegans who did allow use of iodine-enriched sodium chloride.

Therefore, for those individuals with whole-food varied-plant dietary patterns not using iodine-enriched sodium chloride, an iodine supplement is recommended. An example supplement of potassium iodide contains 225 µg[560].

SLEEP SUPPLEMENTS

Perhaps the number one complaint of patients to physicians across all medical specialties is sleep disturbance. There are certainly effective medications available to the prescriber but they are controlled substances and invariably seem to cause tolerance and addiction.

My best advice is to not worry about whether or not you fall asleep, allow it to happen, or not, and be okay with either result.

I recently attended a continuing medical education conference at which a group of physicians were talking about this

A, Rassner S, Akesson B, Ockerman PA (1981) Nutrient intake and health status of vegans. Chemical analyses of diets using the duplicate portion sampling technique. Am J Clin Nutr 34:2464 – 2477.

[559] Waldmann A, Koschizke JW, Leitzmann C, Hahn A 2003 Dietary intakes and lifestyle factors of a vegan population in Germany: results from the German Vegan Study. Eur J Clin Nutr 57:947–955.

[560] As an example, Pure Encapsulations - Iodine (potassium iodide) - Hypoallergenic Supplement contains capsules of 225 µg at a daily cost of $0.12 per capsule.

phenomenon. For those patients really struggling, the suggestion was to use an OTC called Alteril.

Alteril contains "natural" plant extracts, but not in whole-food context. Active ingredients include melatonin, a hormone influencing the sleep-wake cycle that does appear to cross the blood-brain barrier somehow. Each tablet of Alteril contains 2 mg of melatonin. More than a total of about 4 mg tends to cause middle of the night awakening, after the medication is no longer active.

Other ingredients include tryptophan, glycine, skullcap, valerian root, chamomile, hops, and passionflower.

PLANT STANOLS, STEROLS

I hesitated to include this supplement because, although plant derived, stanols and sterols are a concentrated extract. Literature does not indicate side effects from the doses suggested (1.8 grams, see the "portfolio diet") but these have not been examined on a large scale. On the other hand, one of the most prescribed classes of medications in the world for lowering cholesterol, the statins, is known to have a number of side effects[561]. If you have unacceptably high cholesterol counts, are following a strict no-animal-product diet, and do not wish to take a statin drug, this might be an option, particularly in the context of the portfolio diet. Please discuss with your physician.

---

[561] Side effects can include unexplained muscle pain, tenderness, or weakness, confusion, fever, unusual tiredness, and dark colored urine, swelling, weight gain, urinating less than usual or not at all; increased thirst, increased urination, hunger, dry mouth, fruity breath odor, drowsiness, dry skin, blurred vision, weight loss; or nausea, upper stomach pain, itching, loss of appetite, clay-colored stools, jaundice (yellowing of the skin or eyes), diarrhea, or nausea.

As for any of the suggestions in this book, take caution to observe any possible untoward reactions. That is not an easy task and may require a food diary; starting, stopping and starting several times may be required to investigate reactions to a food component or supplement.

Part V HOW

How can one prepare whole-food varied-plant meals to maximize convenience, flavor, and nutrition?

CHAPTER 15

High Temperature Thermal Processing

"Everything in food is science. The only subjective part is when you eat it."

Alton Brown

HIGH TEMPERATURE THERMAL PROCESSING

Thermal processing or "cooking" includes boiling, frying, steaming, baking, microwave heating, and roasting. This can cause biological, physical, and chemical modifications, leading to flavor, nutritional, and textural changes.

Let's throw out frying right away because of the need to use oil extract and the formation of acrylamide, a risk factor for cancer[562].

Otherwise, there are several advantages to cooking that are evident. First, cooking can destroy potentially harmful microorganisms, although in the case of meat, as we have explained, even dead microbes can leave harmful endotoxins. Second, is the enhancement of the digestibility of food and the bioaccessibility of nutrients; for example, the denatured proteins are generally more digestible than native proteins and the gelatinization of starch improves its hydrolysis by amylases.

On the other hand, processing can result in losses of certain nutrients due to chemical reactions, formation of undesired compounds, and loss of desirable texture, flavor, and color.

The three main types of phytochemicals are: carotenoids, glucosinolates and polyphenols. The first two groups include a relatively limited number of compounds compared with the polyphenols. Glucosinolates and polyphenols are soluble in water whereas carotenoids are lipophilic, soluble in oil.

Carotenoids are abundant in yellow–orange fruits and vegetables and in dark green leafy vegetables where often the brilliant colors of the carotenoids are masked by chlorophyll. These colors sometime become apparent in fall temperature changes when the chlorophyll production slows and eventually stops.

When the plant cell wall containing glucosinolates is damaged, the enzyme myrosinase initiates a rapid hydrolysis destroying

---

[562] Stott-Miller, M., Neuhouser, M. L., & Stanford, J. L. (2013). Consumption of deep-fried foods and risk of prostate cancer. *The Prostate, 73*(9), 960-969. doi:10.1002/pros.22643.

glucosinolates. Microwaving, for example, results in sudden collapse of cell structure and myrosinase hydrolyses the glucosinolates[563]. During thermal processing concentrations of glucosinolates can be reduced as a result of enzyme action and thermal breakdown[564]. Boiling results in major loss of glucosinolates through leaching into the hot water[565]. Steaming is the cooking method of choice, although there are still compromises in nutrient reduction.

An analogous situation to the glucosinolates was reported for the polyphenols. Here cell wall rupture invokes polyphenolesterase to inactivate the antioxidants. Leaching and loss into water for this water soluble nutrient class was quite significant. Thus again, steaming was the least destructive cooking method[566].

Depending upon the particular cellular matrix, steaming can result in an *increased* bioaccessibility. This may be by virtue of the breakdown of cellular structures in-situ, without exposure to oxidation or thermal inactivation of oxidative enzymes.

EFFECTS OF THERMAL PROCESSING ON ANTIOXIDANT ACTIVITY OF VEGETABLES

Vegetables contain several hydrophilic (water soluble) and lipophilic (fat soluble) antioxidant compounds and it is important to estimate the antioxidant activity of both as they

---

[563] Palermo, M., Pellegrini, N., & Fogliano, V. (2013). The effect of cooking on the phytochemical content of vegetables. *Journal of the Science of Food and Agriculture, 94*(6), 1057-1070. doi:10.1002/jsfa.6478.

[564] Jones, R., Frisina, C., Winkler, S., Imsic, M., & Tomkins, R. (2010). Cooking method significantly effects glucosinolate content and sulforaphane production in broccoli florets. *Food Chemistry, 123*(2), 237-242. doi:10.1016/j.foodchem.2010.04.016.

[565] Palermo, op cit.

[566] Op cit.

may act together more effectively than singly, synergistically quenching free radicals in both aqueous and lipid phases[567].

One study examined the loss of both hydrophilic and lipophilic antioxidants in a variety of vegetables cooked using boiling, pressure cooking, baking, microwaving, and griddling[568]. The results are shown below.

Figure 20 **Antioxidant Loss in vegetables from cooking, percent**

vegetable	boiling	pressure cook	baking	microwaving	griddling	frying
asparagus	9.1/no loss	9.6/no loss	no loss/no loss	7.4/no loss	9.2/-7.0	8/6.5
beetroot	no loss/5.0	8.2/no ;oss	8/19.6	no loss/22	no loss/no loss	no loss/21.4
broccoli	15.2/32.7	no loss/37.4	no loss/no loss	no loss/34.2	15.9/-6.5	12.2/15.6
cauliflower	32.2/55.0	28.4/36.7	27.4/36.4	10.4/56.7	no loss/11.8	17/23.9
carrot	16.2/33.9	19/43.7	22.5/31.7	no loss/42.2	12.9/13.7	20.1/11.1
garlic	no loss/32.5	no loss/38.9	5.5/19.9	no loss/no loss	6.3/ no loss	no loss/15.5
green beans	no loss/40.0	no loss/25.9	no loss/-12.4	no loss/33.0	11.5/-14.6	7.1/no loss
onion	9.1/no loss	5.3/no loss	no loss/10.1	7/no loss	no loss/-5.6	no loss
peas	14/60.5	12.2/34.5	no loss/38.7	no losss/34.7	12/34.7	17.4/34.6
green peppers	74.8/27.9	72.4/24.5	71.3/no loss	70.4/-9.8	62.2/6.6	24.4/42.9
spinach	30.6/31.6	no loss/18.3	9.7/-6.0	13.5/no loss	17.8/-10.0	19.2/7.8
swiss chard	43/10.8	48.8/no loss	21.7/-8.0	31.3/-6.4	22.6/-10.2	48.1/no loss
zucchini	21.3/51.2	23.3/49.5	16.9/47.5	6.2/36.2	15.6/13.1	20.7/60.9

Note for each vegetable two numbers are given for each cooking method, separated by a right slash; the first number corresponds to the percent loss of hydrophilic antioxidants and the second number the percent loss of lipophilic antioxidants. A negative number indicates a percent increase in nutrient bioaccessibility.

---

[567] Trombino, S., Serini, S., Nicuolo, F. D., Celleno, L., Andò, S., Picci, N., . . . Palozza, P. (2004). Antioxidant Effect of Ferulic Acid in Isolated Membranes and Intact Cells: Synergistic Interactions with α-Tocopherol, β-Carotene, and Ascorbic Acid.*J. Agric. Food Chem. Journal of Agricultural and Food Chemistry, 52*(8), 2411-2420. doi:10.1021/jf0303924.

[568] Jiménez-Monreal, A. M., García-Diz, L., Martínez-Tomé, M., Mariscal, M., & Murcia, M. A. (2009). Influence of Cooking Methods on Antioxidant Activity of Vegetables. *Journal of Food Science, 74*(3). doi:10.1111/j.1750-3841.2009.01091.x.

From the table, it can be seen that boiling results in significant antioxidant loss (asparagus, beetroot, garlic, and onion less so), likely mainly from leaching. Of course, if the water is also consumed, as in soup, the loss is much more favorable (if you don't consume the water, a nice biohack for your garden is to cool the water and pour into your garden soil.)

The antioxidants in cauliflower, carrots, green peppers and zucchini are particularly sensitive to any of the cooking methods examined. On the other hand, asparagus, broccoli, garlic, green beans, onions, and spinach are not very susceptible to thermal degradation, there possibly even being an advantage in the case of griddling (or stir frying) asparagus, broccoli, green beans, and onions.

So in general, cooking at temperatures at or above the boiling point of water has some advantages for safety and digestion but generally results in degradation of nutrient value.

INTRODUCTION TO OTHER VEGETABLE PROCESSING METHODS

In order to provide alternative methods for increasing nutrient bioaccessibility, we shall examine blending, crushing, and lower temperature thermal processing in the following chapters.

CHAPTER 16

Low Temperature Thermal Processing

"All cooking is a matter of time. In general, the more time the better."

John Erskine

DEHYDRATION

Drying is the oldest form of food preservation under the sun, requiring continuous exposure to the sun under non-humid conditions (under about 15% humidity). Food dehydration is a low temperature cooking method that increases the bioaccessibility of plants while intensifying flavor and adding a crisp texture.

These days, electronic food dehydrators use a heat source and air flow to reduce the water content of foods, typically by 80% to 95% for various fruits and vegetables. Most foods are dehydrated at temperatures up to 135 F (57 C). The key to successful food dehydration is the application of a constant low temperature and adequate air flow.

Moisture should be removed as quickly as possible at a temperature that does not significantly adversely affect the nutrition, flavor, and color of the food. Too low a temperature or too long the dehydration time may encourage the growth of bacteria. If the temperature is too high, not only might there be degradation of nutrients but the surface may become hardened with the interior still moist.

Typical home dehydrators have a number of stacked trays; trays can accommodate thin pastes or slices of fruits and vegetables. Most applications will include a variety of fruits and vegetables on various trays. Selection of a typical temperature of 125 F (52 C) then could require the removal of trays at various times depending on the extent of desired dehydration.

Recipe: Kale yes chips

There is obviously no limit to the variety of kale chips that can be made – including just placing raw kale on the dehydrator trays at about 115 F for four hours or so until crispy.

The following is one of my favorite recipes for kale chips[569]. It requires about six lined dehydrator trays (can use without lining, just requires more cleanup).

Start with a good amount of kale, say four bunches. Wash and then strip leaves from the main stem.

---

[569] I have a Nesco professional dehydrator 600W with eight stackable trays and liners.

Ingredients

- 1 cup mixed raw nuts[570]
- 1 cup mixed seeds[571]
- 1 cup garbanzo beans
- 2 tablespoons Braggs Aminos (or soy sauce)
- 2 teaspoons lemon juice
- 3 tablespoons nutritional yeast
- 2 cloves of garlic
- 1 teaspoon turmeric
- 2 pinches of black ground pepper

Instructions

- Place all ingredients into high speed blender for 30 seconds.
- Add water until the consistency is similar to hummus.
- Transfer the blender contents into a large mixing bowl, lining the edges with the mixture.
- Begin adding kale and knead into the mixture.
- Continue until all the kale has been added and uniformly coated with the mixture.
- Add the coated kale to the lined trays.
- Power on for 6 hours or more at 125 F (52 C) until crisp.

This batch is more than you or your family will eat at one sitting. Dehydrated foods rehydrate rather quickly, so depending upon the environment, placing into ziplock bags (gallon size) is a good idea. I usually place into vacuum bags and evacuate air for storage in the refrigerator or freezer.

---

[570] I use *Food to Live* Mixed Raw Nuts (Cashews, Brazil Nuts, Walnuts, Almonds).

[571] I use *Gerbs'* Pumpkin, Sunflower, Chia, Flax, Hemp Seed Raw Mix.

SOUS VIDE

Sous vide is French for "under vacuum" and sous vide cooking is defined as

> *"foods that are cooked under controlled conditions of temperature and time inside heat-stable vacuumed pouches[572]".*

Sous vide cooking differs from traditional cooking methods in at least four main ways: the raw food is vacuum-sealed in heat-stable, food-grade plastic pouches and cooked using precisely controlled heating (within 0.1 C); lower temperatures and longer cooking times are used.

Vacuum sealing has several benefits: it increases the food's shelf life by eliminating the risk of recontamination by aerobic bacteria during storage; inhibits poor flavors that result from oxidation; and prevents evaporative losses of flavor volatiles and moisture during cooking resulting in delicious and nutritious food[573].

The close control of temperature allows for excellent reproducibility of recipes. Because of the close proximity of the contacting surface of the vegetable with the heating water and the longer contact times, the degree of cooking is equal throughout the item, from surface to interior.

---

[572] Schellekens, M. (1996). New research issues in sous-vide cooking. *Trends in Food Science & Technology, 7*(8), 256-262. doi:10.1016/0924-2244(96)10027-3.

[573] Church, I. J., & Parsons, A. L. (2000). The sensory quality of chicken and potato products prepared using cook-chill and sous vide methods. *International Journal of Food Science and Technology, 35*(2), 155-162. doi:10.1046/j.1365-2621.2000.00361.x.

Sous vide low temperature thermal processing can reduce the nutrient losses caused by high temperature cooking methods. Sous-vide cooking of vegetables is performed at temperatures of about 185 F (85 C) in order to break-down the intercellular material[574] and soften the individual cell walls[575].

During traditional cooking of green vegetables, for example, bright green colors turn olive green due to the degradation of chlorophyll, caused by the loss of the central magnesium atom[576]. By cooking at temperatures lower than 100 C, the thermal degradation of chlorophyll is reduced.

In the case of phytonutrients such as carotenoids, which are vulnerable to oxidation and degradation by heat, reduced exposure to oxygen during sous-vide cooking improves nutrient retention[577]. Thus, sous-vide cooked vegetables retain higher levels of antioxidant activity and antioxidant compounds (total polyphenols, vitamin C and carotenoids) than other higher temperature cooking techniques[578]. Compared to traditional

---

[574] The intercellular connecting material is called the middle lamella, a substance that acts as a cementing material between the cell walls of adjacent cells. The middle lamella is composed of pectin, cellulose, calcium and other polymers.

[575] Sila, D. N., Doungla, E., Smout, C., Loey, A. V., & Hendrickx, M. (2006). Pectin Fraction Interconversions: Insight into Understanding Texture Evolution of Thermally Processed Carrots. *J. Agric. Food Chem. Journal of Agricultural and Food Chemistry, 54*(22), 8471-8479. doi:10.1021/ jf0613379.

[576] Damodaran, S., Parkin, K.L., & Fennema, O.R. (2008). Fennema's Food Chemistry. (4th ed.). Boca Raton, FL: CRC Press.

[577] Chiavaro, E., Mazzeo, T., Visconti, A., Manzi, C., Fogliano, V., & Pellegrini, N. (2012). Nutritional quality of sous vide cooked carrots and Brussels Sprouts. Journal of Agricultural and Food Chemistry, 60, 6019–6025.

[578] Baardseth, P., Bjerke, F., Martinsena, B. K., & Skredea, G. (2010). Vitamin C, total phenolics and antioxidative activity in tip-cut green beans (Phaseolus vulgaris) and swede rods (Brassica napus var. napo-

cooking, sous vide cooking of vegetables also reduces the degradation of a variety of other phytonutrients[579] [580].

SOUS VIDE SETUP

I use a first generation 800 W Anova Precision Cooker with Wi-Fi control shown here. I attach the unit to the side of a large pasta pot with the attachment device that comes with the sous vide cooker. It works by forced circulation and an enclosed heating element.

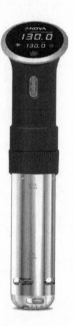

I use vacuum bags that are free of BPA, phthalates, and other plasticizers. It's the *plasticizers* – chemical additives like phthalates that increase the pliability and fluidity of the plastic – that contain estrogenic activity.

I place the vegetables of interest into the bags and evacuate using a vacuum sealing system[581]. I then place the bags into the pasta pot and assure that they remain submerged using office-type binder clips.

---

brassica) processed by methods used in catering. Journal of the Science and Food Agriculture, 90, 1245–1255.

[579] Stea, T. H., Johansson, M., Jägerstad, M., & Frølich, W. (2007). Retention of folates in cooked, stored and reheated peas, broccoli and potatoes for use in modern large-scale service systems. *Food Chemistry, 101*(3), 1095-1107. doi:10.1016/j.foodchem.2006.03.009.

[580] Chiavaro, E., Mazzeo, T., Visconti, A., Manzi, C., Fogliano, V., & Pellegrini, N. (2012). Nutritional Quality of Sous Vide Cooked Carrots and Brussels Sprouts. *J. Agric. Food Chem. Journal of Agricultural and Food Chemistry, 60*(23), 6019-6025. doi:10.1021/jf300692a.

[581] I have a FoodSaver V2244 Vacuum Sealing System.

Virtually any vegetable can be selected for sous vide cooking. From Table 20, particularly excellent candidates would be those vegetables that are degraded most from high temperature cooking, such as cauliflower, carrots, green peppers, and zucchini. Green leaves can be processed with little nutrient loss or color change.

Recipe: Sous Vide Ratatouille *Niçoise*

This recipe utilizes zucchini and green peppers, sensitive to high-temperature cooking. Makes enough for about 4 people.

Ingredients

- 1 medium size zucchini, quartered lengthwise, and cut into one half inch pieces
- 1 medium size eggplant, cut into 1/2-inch pieces (about 2 - 3 cups)
- 1 red bell pepper, chopped
- 1 onion, chopped
- 1 cup tomatoes, chopped course
- 2 garlic cloves, minced
- ½ cup shredded fresh basil leaves
- ¼ teaspoon oregano
- ¼ teaspoon thyme or coriander

Instructions

- Set the sous vide cooker for 185 F (85 C)
- Put the zucchini, tomatoes, bell peppers, eggplant, and onion each in its own vacuum seal bag.
- Distribute the garlic and basil equally amongst each bag.
- Vacuum seal each bag.

- Once the water has reached the set-point temperature, submerge each bag.
- Set a timer for 30 minutes; once that time is up, remove the tomatoes.
- Set the timer for 30 more minutes; once that time is up, remove the zucchini and peppers.
- Set the timer for one hour; once that time is up, remove the eggplant and onion.
- Mix the contents of each bag into a large serving bowl; season with black pepper to taste.

CHAPTER 17

Mechanical Processing

"If you think well, you cook well."
Ferran Adria

BLENDING: A TORNADO IN THE KITCHEN

The high speed blender is the key kitchen tool for assuring intake of nutrients vital to physical and mental health. When I make a "smoothie," aptly named because the contents are either solubilized or micron-size particles suspended in water giving a smooth appearance, I am less concerned about the taste than the nutrition. This is a particularly terrific way to process green leafy vegetables, hence the oft-used term "green smoothie." The blender does the "chewing," so that more of this most nutritious of all food groups can be consumed.

Green leafy plants generally have a very high nutrient to calorie ratio. This is related to the high surface to volume ratio in leaves – the sun's energy is more available for nutrient

333

manufacture. However, in general leaves are rather tough and bitter, a protective defense developed by immobile plants. That's a tough reality as the leaves of plants can provide an excellent variety of macronutrients, vitamins and minerals, and a vast array of phytonutrients.

I have found it difficult to eat more than about one pound of leaves per day (that is equal to about seven cups of raw chopped kale, for example, providing about 200 calories). This is partly because gathering time from the garden is significant and storage is rather a problem unless you shop every few days. So, as much as you like the idea of being "powered by kale" energetically (calorically), it ain't gonna happen.

Luckily, we don't have to rely on leaves for our entire energy source; that would take a great deal of chewing time, although that is precisely what our primate ancestors did for nearly 85 million years[582] and other primates do today.

As those in Western civilization do not allocate much time for green leaf chewing, how *can* one consume a significant amount of this optimal food source? The answer is food processing to assist with the chewing: smashing between stones (as mortar and pestle), cooking (laying in the sun, roasting, baking, boiling, etc.) or my favorite choice: high speed blending.

My smoothies taste nutritious if not delicious. I don't obsess about the taste but if unsatisfactory, additional fruit will improve the bitter-to-sweet ratio. A single ripe date can often be enough to increase palatability to more acceptable levels.

---

[582] Aiken, R.C. & Aiken, D.C. (2015), The New Ancestral Diet, Go Ahead Publishing.

BIOACCESSIBILITY

Besides the function of hiding the bitter tastes of superfoods and allowing us to eat parts of plants we wouldn't ordinarily eat – such as citrus peels and seeds - the complete disruption of the rigid cellulose plant cell walls makes available cellular contents more *bioaccessible*.

It's not enough to have high nutrient concentration; it is just as important that the nutrients are bioaccessible. In order to be accessible for absorption in the gut, the nutrients have to be released from the food matrix[583]. Nutrient bioavailability additionally includes nutrient absorption, metabolism, tissue distribution and bioactivity[584]. This means that a prerequisite for nutrient bioavailability is its bioaccessibility.

For example, it has been shown that only particles smaller than the size of an individual cell can result in high carotenoid bioaccessibility, and that cell wall destruction is an important prerequisite for carotenoids to be released from the plant particles to enhance bioavailability[585]. Typical plant cells have a size ranging from 10 – 100 microns, while chewing results in

---

[583] Faulks, R. M., & Southon, S. (2005). Challenges to understanding and measuring carotenoid bioavailability. *Biochimica Et Biophysica Acta (BBA) - Molecular Basis of Disease, 1740*(2), 95-100. doi:10.1016/j.bbadis.2004.11.012.

[584] Parada, J., & Aguilera, J. (2007). Food Microstructure Affects the Bioavailability of Several Nutrients. *Journal of Food Science J Food Science, 72*(2). doi:10.1111/j.1750-3841.2007.00274.x.

[585] Moelants, K. R., Lemmens, L., Vandebroeck, M., Buggenhout, S. V., Loey, A. M., & Hendrickx, M. E. (2012). Relation between Particle Size and Carotenoid Bioaccessibility in Carrot- and Tomato-Derived Suspensions. *J. Agric. Food Chem. Journal of Agricultural and Food Chemistry, 60*(48), 11995-12003. doi:10.1021/jf303502h.

particle size distributions with means in the thousands of microns[586] (with an average of 10 chews per bite).

This is probably the case for many foods and many nutrients.

Here's how it's done physically.

BLENDER MECHANICAL PROPERTIES

There are two primary physical processes that work to mechanically break down the cell wall of plants, releasing nutrients: shear forces and cavitation.

Shear forces are created by the high-speed impact of the food with the blender blades. This includes direct cutting by the blade itself as well as shearing by application of high kinetic energy of the particulate matter moving through the surrounding medium and striking other particles and the container. But the real powerful action is cavitation.

Cavitation is caused by the Bernoulli effect – the same principle behind air flight – planes and helicopters, and why boats can sail faster against the wind than with the wind. The speed of the blades in fluid cause a decrease in pressure above the blades equal to the vapor pressure of the fluid, similar to boiling. Bubbles form on the blades (assuming a fluid component), are flung away and implode causing very powerful shockwaves that further break down even the smallest of remaining particles.

---

[586] Bornhorst, G. M., & Singh, R. P. (2012). Bolus Formation and Disintegration during Digestion of Food Carbohydrates. *Comprehensive Reviews in Food Science and Food Safety, 11*(2), 101-118. doi:10.1111/j.1541-4337.2011.00172.x.

OXIDATION

In essence, high speed blenders (1.5 horsepower or greater) create a food tornado with a low pressure core that rapidly sucks in air – at 20% oxygen – into the mix. That's not good for antioxidants: we want them to do their oxidation duties in our bodies, not be oxidized in the blender.

So are blenders bad to use for this reason? Read on.

Polyphenoloxidases (PPO)

The enzymes in the class PPO appear to reside in the plastids (small organelles in the cytoplasm of plant cells) of all plants and are released when the plastid cell membrane is disrupted. PPO is thought to play an important role in the resistance of plants to microbial and viral infections and to adverse climatic conditions.

Phenolic compounds are responsible for the color of many plants and impart taste and flavor. They are very important antioxidants.

In the presence of oxygen from air, the PPO enzyme catalyzes the first steps in the biochemical conversion of phenolics to produce quinones, which undergo further polymerization to yield dark, insoluble polymers referred to as melanin. This is the same melanin that determines darkness of human skin and hair. In plants, melanin forms barriers and has antimicrobial properties that prevent the spread of infection in plant tissues.

Note that enzymatic browning is considered desirable for the color and taste of tea, coffee, and chocolate. You have witnessed this in many fruits and vegetables as the darkening of a cut surface of apples, bananas, and avocados as examples.

Phenolic substances in plants

Phenolic compounds are one of the few main groupings of phytonutrients. There are many phenolic (or polyphenolic) compounds in fruits and vegetables, all water soluble. Epidemiological studies and associated meta-analyses strongly suggest that long-term consumption of diets rich in plant polyphenols offers protection against development of cancers, vascular diseases, diabetes, osteoporosis, psychiatric and neurodegenerative diseases[587].

Polyphenols can be divided into many different subcategories, such as anthocyans, flavanols, curcuminoids and flavonoids. Flavonoids are formed in plants from the aromatic amino acids phenylalanine and tyrosine. Tyrosine also synthesizes DOPA (3,4-dihydroxyphenethylamine) that forms dopamine.

Many plants synthesize dopamine to varying degrees. The highest concentrations have been observed in bananas, levels of 40 to 50 parts per million by weight. I mention this because I selected bananas to study experimentally antioxidant loss in high-speed blending.

Effect of acidity

The optimum pH for PPO activity has been shown to be 7 (dopamine substrate). However, the enzyme displays high activity between pH 6.5–7.5 and the activity rapidly decreases at more acidic pH values[588].

---

[587] Pandey, K. B., & Rizvi, S. I. (2009). Plant Polyphenols as Dietary Antioxidants in Human Health and Disease. *Oxidative Medicine and Cellular Longevity, 2*(5), 270-278. doi:10.4161/oxim.2.5.9498.

[588] Chaisakdanugull, C., and Theerakulkait, C. (2009) Partial purification and characterization of banana [Musa (AAA Group) 'Gros Michel'] polyphenol oxidase, International J of Food Science and Technology 44, 840-846.

Effect of temperature on PPO stability

Heating at 60 C for 30 minutes reduces the enzymatic activity by 50%; heating at 90 C completely destroys the enzyme. The optimum temperature for maximum activity is 30 C (86 F). Unfortunately, heating not only destroys the PPO, it can also degrade the phytonutrients.

Chemical Inhibition of PPO

It has been shown that complete inhibition of PPO activity is found with as low as 0.8 millimolar (mm) ascorbic acid[589]. Ascorbic acid, also known as vitamin C, acts as an antioxidant because it reduces the initial quinone formed by the enzyme to the original diphenol.

Citric acid also can inhibit PPO activity, although not as strongly as ascorbic acid[590]. Citric acid exists in much greater than trace amounts in a variety of fruits and vegetables, most notably citrus fruits. Lemons and limes have particularly high concentrations of the acid; it can constitute as much as 8% of the dry weight of these fruits. The concentrations of citric acid in citrus fruits range from 0.005 mol/L for oranges and grapefruits to 0.30 mol/L in lemons and limes[591].

---

[589] Ünal, M. Ü. (2007). Properties of polyphenol oxidase from Anamur banana (Musa cavendishii). *Food Chemistry, 100*(3), 909-913. doi:10.1016/ j.foodchem.2005.10.048.

[590] Yang, C., Fujita, S., Ashrafuzzaman, M., Nakamura, N., & Hayashi, N. (2000). Purification and Characterization of Polyphenol Oxidase from Banana (Musa sapientum L .) Pulp. *J. Agric. Food Chem. Journal of Agricultural and Food Chemistry, 48*(7), 2732-2735. doi:10.1021/jf991037.

[591] Penniston KL, Nakada SY, Holmes RP, Assimos DG; Nakada; Holmes; Assimos (2008). "Quantitative Assessment of Citric Acid in Lemon Juice, Lime Juice, and Commercially-Available Fruit Juice Products" *.Journal of Endourology* 22 (3): 567–570.

Experiment

I conducted a very simple experiment[592] to access the effects of acidity, ascorbic acid and citric acid content, pH, and temperature on the degree of oxidation of the polyphenols in bananas versus blending speed and blending time. The results were surprising.

The juice of one small lime was enough to effectively stop polyphenol oxidation, even at the highest blending speeds for prolonged blending times; temperature had little effect. While this was a very simple experiment with bananas,

> *When using high-speed blending, toss in a whole lime or lemon in water or ice and blend that first. Then add other ingredients and blend.*

there is reason to believe the chemistry would be similar for other antioxidants in fruits and vegetables.

Smoothie recipe for health and happiness

First gather fresh local fruits and vegetables. However, I find that for regular smoothie preparation (almost daily in my household), I simply cannot keep a continuous fresh source available. I solve that dilemma by purchasing fresh frozen organic mixtures of fruits and vegetables.

The fruits I typically use are a mixture of organic frozen strawberries, blackberries, and blueberries from Chile and marketed by Cascadian Farms; package contents are 10 oz. (284 gm) so about enough for two cups – I use one cup per

---

[592] Details with photos and videos on this experiment can be found on our website www.moodforlife.com. Search terms blender and bio-hack. Here is the url: http://moodforlife.com/index.php/minimization-oxidation-reaction-high-speed-blending/.

smoothie. I try to always have a berry source and these mixed berries cover that need quite well.

The organic frozen vegetables are from the same distributor, consisting of broccoli, cauliflower, carrots, and zucchini. Again one package is 10 oz. (284 gm) and makes two cups, one of which I use for each smoothie. I like this mixture as it contains two cruciferous vegetables. Of course, any fresh organic source of vegetables on hand can substitute for the frozen.

There is more limited availability of fresh organic frozen greens. We have a garden that is primarily reserved for green leafy vegetables. Kale and mint grow year-round even in our cold Missouri winters without any extra effort on our part. However, most varieties of greens must be obtained from the grocery store during the wintry months.

FREEZING GREENS

To avoid frequent trips to the store to replenish a fresh supply of greens, one can freeze them, at least for use in smoothies where a little withering and icing of the produce doesn't matter.

Greens may be available in your store - organic, prewashed in a container; if so, and you can afford it, buy that. I hesitate buying any food, leaves in particular (high surface area) that are on the shelves open to general handling (organic or otherwise). However, if you do, a thorough washing/ decontamination is warranted.

Remove all stems (stems usually are not very nutrient rich and tend to give an unwanted stringy texture to smoothies).

After washing your hands thoroughly, wash leaves in water. This can be a little time consuming, but if done for a bulk of leaves, the process is more time efficient. Place washed leaves in a large salad spinner[593] to remove most of the water.

Decontaminate. I use a homemade vegetable wash solution consisting of 1:1 apple vinegar to tap water and two tablespoons of lemon or lime juice in a 16 oz. spray bottle[594]. Spray each leaf. These can once again be spun to remove excess solution or simply placed into the plastic storage bag. I like the citrus coating to assist reduction of oxidation, as detailed above.

I recommend when preparing any food for the freezer, that a vacuum sealer be used to reduce the oxidation (See Chapter 16). I typically make about a dozen quart-sized bags (each equivalent to three to four cups of greens).

Super smoothie

My smoothie recipe has lots of fresh or frozen green leaves, frozen organic fruits and vegetables as the base and several added "superfoods." As the preparation of this can still be time consuming if done individually, I make a dozen or so preparations at a time, vacuum seal and freeze.

Here is a step-by-step example.

- Place one quartered lemon or lime into your high-speed blender (I use a Vitamix Turboblend VS) with ice or water and blend until well mixed.
- Add three or four cups of fresh or frozen mixture of green leafy vegetables.

---

[593] I use an OXO "good grips" that measures 7.5 inches x 10.5 inches x 10.5 inches and costs under $30.

[594] For example Soft 'N Style 6 bottles for under $12.

- Add one cup vegetables, including cruciferous, into the blender. For example, the above referenced frozen Cascadian Farms organic broccoli, cauliflower, carrots, and zucchini.
- Add one cup of fruit, including berries, into the blender. For example, one half of the above referenced frozen Cascadian Farms organic frozen strawberries, blackberries, and blueberries.
- Add one heaping tablespoon flaxseed.
- Add one teaspoon turmeric and fresh ground black pepper.
- Add other nutraceutics from your potion shelf. I usually include a variety of herbs and spices such as those listed in Chapter 14.
- Add additional water to fill most of the blender (50 of the 64 ounce capacity).
- Blend for 30 – 60 seconds.
- Taste test. If too bitter, sweeten with additional fruit; dates are very sweet and very nutritious. One to two dates usually makes the difference.

Sip and swirl

There are certain chemical reactions associated with digestion that occur in the mouth, so it is a good idea to allow sufficient contact time in the mouth for that to occur. The other reason to "sip" is to give the gastrointestinal system time to respond to the food input and achieve an appropriate degree of satiation; otherwise, one may be inclined to supplement the smoothie with less healthy food.

I like to drink a 12-ounce glass slowly, then take a 28-ounce Blender Bottle with me to work or play to sip during the day. I might take swallows between patients, for example. This "biohack" keeps hunger at bay and provides energy and nutrients at a "slow-released" rate that allows for improved bioavailability.

CRUSHING: THE STONE AGE WAY

I do appreciate texture, so there are certain vegetables that I rarely blend but rather consume in a different manner. These include underground storage organs (USOs) such as sweet potatoes, onions, and garlic; also beans and grains.

I try to include *lots* of green leafy vegetables with every meal. Blending is one way to mechanically chew but another method yields a nice texture to USOs, grains, and beans: stone crushing.

This was possibly the first food processing technique, originating in the Stone Age, namely crushing plants between two stones. I use the mortar and pestle shown below.

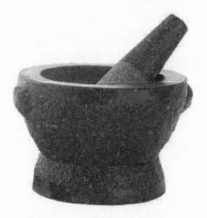

This is a 3+ cup capacity 8-inch diameter stone from a single block of granite. It is practically indestructible – will not chip or crack even under vigorous pounding (Mohs scale 7+). It's also beautiful[595].

---

[595] From Thailand; cost was $34 online on Amazon.

My initial use was specifically for making pesto using basil, garlic, walnuts, and nutritional yeast. However, now its use has expanded to a variety of pestos or pastes.

I recommend a home garden if you have any land at all. Even a balcony can provide a vertical garden. Even with no land or balcony, various seeds can be sprouted for a fast, fresh, organic, nutritious, continuous harvest.

Much of what is grown we start from seeds. We use heritage seeds from Baker Creek Heirloom Seed Company[596].

Stone Age Buddha Bowl

The first ingredient extracted from our garden was kale. Each ingredient was weighed so as to provide a precise nutritional summary. Below is the scale weighting a portion of the kale, 17 grams worth.

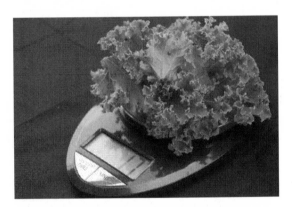

The total amount of kale used, 130 grams, is shown below in the mortar. On the left before crushing and on the right, after exactly five minutes of crushing. You can see the tough leaves are considerably reduced in volume to a paste.

---

[596] The largest online heirloom seed company in the United States and coincidently located just down the street from our ranch near Mansfield, Missouri, home of *Little House on the Prairie* author Laura Ingalls Wilder.

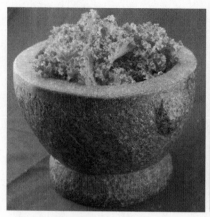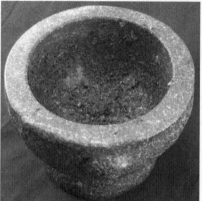

Next from our garden came arugula, 25 gm; greens from the heritage beet plant "Early Wonder", pre-1811, 41 gm; basil, 26 gm; and dandelion, 12 gm[597].

Also added to the mortar were garlic cloves, 16 grams; flaxseed, 4 grams; freshly crushed black pepper, 0.5 grams; and a slice of lemon with peel, 23 grams.

These ingredients were crushed for about seven minutes. Next, freshly sprouted buckwheat, 64 grams, was added.

Organically grown black beans were soaked in water overnight to begin the sprouting process, then slowly cooked the previous day. I used about one and a half cups, 245 grams.

This recipe provides two servings, one is shown below. I call this my "Buddha Bowl," or, alternatively here in the Ozarks, my "Bubba Bowl[598]". The texture is wonderful. A tablespoon of flaxseeds is a

---

[597] The dandelion greens are from a single plant; ironically our lawn is maintained by a service that apparently uses chemicals that discourage "weeds". This sole dandelion was found growing in a flowerpot of Missouri Primrose.

[598] See our Facebook Page "The Hillbilly Vegan".

nice accompaniment. Favorite spices can be added such as turmeric and black pepper.

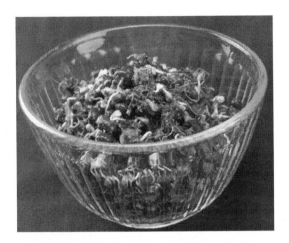

Analysis

The total weight of this combination of food is 592.5 gm; it results in 648.2 calories. The breakdown in calories are:

- carbohydrates: 71%
- protein: 19%
- fat: 10%

This is close to the ideal caloric distribution given in Chapter 12; it is a little higher in protein because of the black beans. There are 31.8 grams of fiber, 3.0 grams of omega-3, and 1.7 grams of omega-6.

Most importantly, it is very high in phytonutrients.

CHAPTER 18

Special Occasions

"I love Thanksgiving because it's a holiday that is centered around food and family, two things that are of utmost importance to me."

Marcus Samuelsson

ROASTING AND COOKING OVER AN OPEN FIRE

While we try to minimize high temperature cooking, on special occasions we allow exceptions. The following details a special whole-food varied-plant Thanksgiving meal tradition.

SACRED FOUR-DIRECTIONS HARVEST TABLE VEGAN THANKSGIVING

It seems appropriate for Thanksgiving celebrations to adopt the Cherokee Plant Medicine teachings and traditions honoring indigenous ways of balance and respect for the earth, the sacred four-directions harvest table.

Our harvest table shown below is eight feet long and about three feet wide; the length was chosen as equal to the length of the hearth and the opening of the firebox of our fireplace. It is sufficiently long so that several persons can sit along the one side – on a bench – looking into the fire, providing light and warmth to the body and heart. The top consists of three planks. The outer two planks are about a foot wide, wide enough for one plate to seat squarely.

The heart of the harvest table is the middle plank. One blustery spring day, we approached our cabin to discover that our favorite tree, a splendid walnut, had toppled. There it lay in repose for over a year until it occurred to us that we could give it new life as the middle plank in our harvest table.

The rest of the table is from oak trees similarly selected by strong winds and milled by a friend not far from the property.

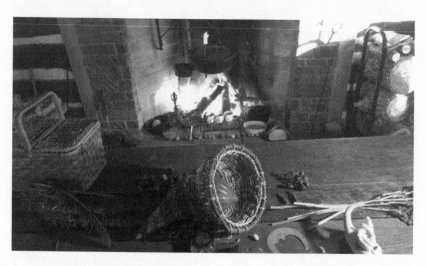

THE CELEBRATION

First identify the four directions. We selected the site for our log cabin and laid out the main pen to face due magnetic north so the directions of each side of the room and the table are true.

The cornucopia is placed in the center of the table with items of nourishment, fruit and vegetables. For the four directions, choose objects and colors that relate to the energies of each direction. These could be edible, but not necessarily.

East: Red or yellow to represent the sun; importance of family life; importance of women as Mother Earth, those who give life; importance of the heart in relationships and life. We choose a red heart of alabaster (sun, fire, love), red holly berries and leaves (fertility, mother), red and yellow heirloom tomatoes, dandelion leaves, dried cayenne peppers, and the Buddha's hand (citrus).

South: White or green; exposure to nature; innocence; the child who learns. Represented by antique mother-of-pearl tie clasp, ivy sprigs, green-white squash, rosemary, a goose feather, a white paper cutting of deer and fir trees, a small tin handcrafted angel with inscription "No man is a failure who has friends".

West: Black to represent sacredness or the "darkening land"- the setting of the sun and the protection of the moon. We represented these ideas with blackened freshly fallen whole walnuts, dark heirloom tomato, dark purple grapes, and coffee beans.

North: Sky blue, dark blue, purple, or sometimes white to represent the sky and the snow of the North. The four winds, cold weather, calm. The adult who teaches. We offered a

Native American turquoise and silver bracelet, mint, Thuja sprigs, chestnuts, sage, and a folk art tin moon.

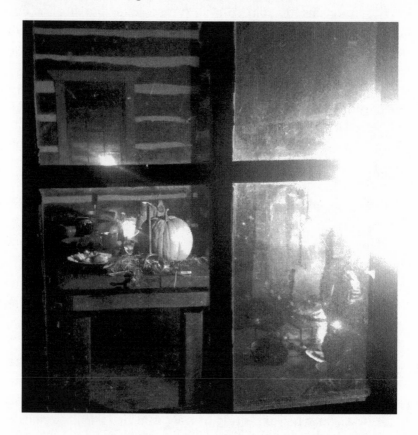

Recipe: Sacred Four-Directions Harvest Thanksgiving Stew

- Place a dozen or so new potatoes on the hearth close to the fire; turn once in a while.
- Place a dozen small onions or shallots on the hearth with the potatoes, also turning.
- Place sliced bell peppers, green and red, into a trivet and place over glowing ashes.
- Place a loaf of freshly baked sourdough bread on the hearth, also turning occasionally.

- Place peeled garlic cloves into a small iron skillet directly on the glowing ashes.

Enjoy the hearth fire and company. Once the potatoes and onions are soft, the peppers slightly scorched, and the garlic buttery, cut the potatoes, onions, and peppers and put into a large Dutch oven. Spoon in the garlic, mashed. To this add:

- 1 28-ounce can diced tomatoes
- 1 cup vegetable broth
- 1 large can black beans or chili beans
- 1/2 teaspoon ground black pepper
- zest of lemon peel and juice of one lemon
- 1 cup finely chopped greens
- favorite spices to taste

Sir well and place Dutch oven on fireplace crane over glowing hardwood logs; let simmer for an hour or two, stirring occasionally with a large ladle.

When complete, ladle generously into bowls and serve with toasted sourdough bread.

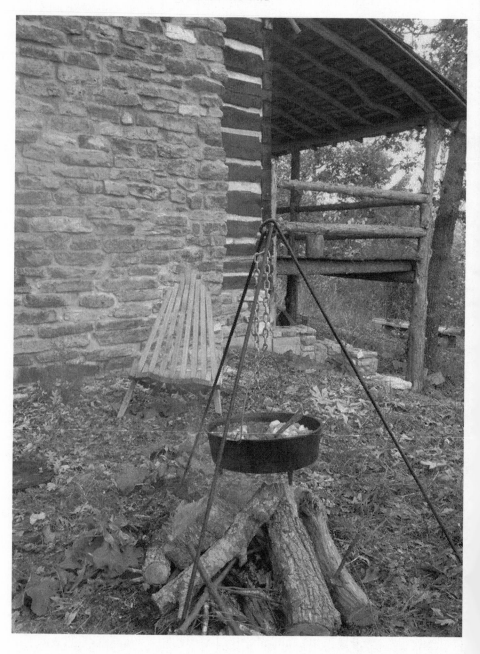

CHAPTER 19

Changing Habits using Cognitive Behavioral Therapy

"There is nothing either good or bad, but thinking makes it so."

William Shakespeare, Hamlet, Act 2, Scene 2

HOW TO CHANGE YOUR DIETARY PATTERN

This book has detailed the emergence of cognitive and emotional dysfunction related to Western dietary changes. I have included extensive peer-reviewed scientific studies to support my claim of the great benefits of a whole-food varied-plant diet. My thinking is that if one *knows* that a certain dietary/ behavioral pattern is vital to their health and happiness, they are more likely to follow it.

However, there may be a number of other lifestyle choices that one knows are important, but one does not follow - a few examples being exercise, spirituality, taking time to develop relationships and having healthy fun. So how does one begin to incorporate important new behavior until it is a habit, a lifestyle?

That is what the current chapter is all about.

WHAT IS YOUR WHY

In order to reach a goal of a smart dietary pattern, one must have reasons behind it that are consistently and consciously understood. Some possible whys are:

- I want to optimize my physical, cognitive, and emotional self.
- I want to avoid physical, cognitive, and emotional problems.
- I want to treat my current physical, cognitive, or emotional problems.
- I want to live ethically and morally, not encouraging the cruelty or murder of animals.
- I want to lose weight.
- I want to look better and feel better.

The key is changing the way you think.

COGNITIVE BEHAVIORAL THERAPY: IT'S THE THOUGHT THAT COUNTS

Cognitive-Behavioral Therapy (CBT) is a form of psychotherapy that emphasizes the important role of thinking in how we feel and what we do. It suggests that it is our thinking that causes us to feel and act the way we do. Therefore, if we are experiencing unwanted feelings and behaviors, it is important to identify the associated thinking and to learn how to replace this thinking with thoughts that lead to more desirable results. We shall use the following definition of CBT:

> *CBT is an active, brief form of therapy or therapeutic intervention that focuses on a person changing dysfunctional or irrational thoughts, leading to more positive emotions and behaviors.*

No one "makes" us think one way or another or has control over our emotions and behavior. We can think in ways consistent with our goals or not, our choice - the former is healthy, the latter unhealthy.

We develop "cognitive schemata" over time that integrates experience into basic beliefs. These schemata develop early in life, become reinforced over time, and are consolidated by adulthood. It is the aim of CBT to uncover these schemata or core beliefs, examine them, and make any useful changes by an active involvement.

If your dietary pattern has heretofore not been a part of your cognitive, emotional, or ethical portfolio, you may have established ways of thinking that need to be re-examined.

INTRODUCTION

There are several approaches to cognitive-behavioral therapy, but most cognitive-behavioral therapies have the following characteristics:

- CBT states that our thoughts cause our feelings and be-haviors, not situations. We can change the way we think and therefore the way we feel and act regardless of the situation.

- CBT is based on the here and now and does not require an understanding of "how you got there", although identification of "core beliefs" assists long-lasting growth.

- CBT is reality based. The idea is that if we can understand a situation for what it really is, rather than as viewed through distorted conditioned responses, we can better deal with it.

COGNITIVE AND BEHAVIORAL THERAPIES

Cognitive behavioral therapy combines two effective kinds of psychotherapy — cognitive therapy and behavior therapy.

Behavior therapy helps you weaken the connections between troublesome situations and your habitual reactions to them. It also teaches you how to calm your mind and body, so you can feel better, think more clearly, and make better decisions.

Mark Twain once said that *"Life is just mind over matter: if you don't mind, it doesn't matter."* The inversion of that thought is that if you do mind, then it does matter. Let your dietary pattern matter.

Cognitive therapy teaches you how certain thinking patterns are causing your symptoms by giving you a distorted picture of what's going on in your life and resulting in negative feelings such as anxiety, sadness, or anger without basis in reality.

WHY USE CBT?

CBT has been studied more than any other psychotherapy and is the only evidence-based effective treatment for a variety of emotional/ behavioral adjustments. Many controlled research studies indicate its effectiveness in a variety of settings.

SOCRATIC QUESTIONING

CBT has philosophic roots in the work of Socrates. The story of Socrates is well known: he traveled through the city of Athens talking with many notable citizens of the day and questioning their views.

A similar approach[599] [600] is used with CBT in that the individual needs to note and examine negative "self-talk" and logically examine these thoughts through a series of questions such as the following:

- *Why do you think that is right?*
- *What led you to think that?*
- *How did you come to that conclusion?*
- *Are those good enough reasons?*
- *What's another way to think about it?*

The following table includes some ideas.

---

[599] Overholser, J. C. (1993). "Elements of the Socratic method: II. Inductive reasoning". *Psychotherapy* 30: 75–85.

[600] Overholser, J. C. (1994). "Elements of the Socratic method: III. Universal definitions". *Psychotherapy* 31 (2): 286–293.

Figure 21 Questions that Probe Reason and Evidence

Questions of Clarification	Questions that Probe Assumptions	Questions that Probe Reason and Evidence
What is the meaning of that?	What am I assuming?	What would be an example?
What's my main point?	Why do I think that holds true here?	How do I know?
Let me see if I understand; do I mean ___ or ___ ?	Am I sure? Am I afraid that is true or know it to be a fact?	Do I have any evidence for that?
Could I give an example?	What else could I assume instead?	By what reasoning did I come to that conclusion?

THE CBT MODEL OF THE HUMAN EXPERIENCE

A simple model of the human experience is the following: a trigger ("T"), usually from the external environment, results in an automatic thought ("AT"). The thought leads to an associated emotion ("E") that in turns can result in a behavioral response ("R"). Putting these elements together spells the acronym TATER, illustrated here[601].

---

[601] We have published a workbook titled "Think Again" (Aiken, R.C., Go Ahead Publishing, 2016) that utilizes this TATER acronym as a playful theme to teach the basic aspects of CBT to adolescents and young adults. The workbook can be used standalone, or in individual or group therapy. Although geared to younger adults and adolescents, it can be effectively used by older adults as well.

T is for Trigger

Triggers can be big or small,
    good or bad or in-between.

AT is for Automatic Thought

This is the first thought that
comes into your head.

E is for Emotion

The way you feel follows the way
you think.

R is for Response

This is what actions you take, your
behavior.

TRIGGER HAPPY

You follow this pattern continuously through out the day, although you may be unaware of it. Triggers can be very small, very large, or in-between. They can be based on biology, ecology, or psychology and lead to automatic thoughts.

Some triggers/ automatic thoughts based on biology:

- "I feel hungry and need to eat – anything, now."
- "I don't feel full – I need to feel full in order to be satisfied."
- "I love the taste of (an unhealthy food) and my body craves it."
- "I have to eat only very tasty food every meal."

Some triggers/ automatic thoughts based on ecology (your environment):

- At the supermarket: "This looks so good, I'll make this one exception."
- At home, if it's in your house, it's in your mouth[602].
- At a friend's house, "I just want to be friendly."
- "When I travel, there is no other choice but to eat poorly."
- "I'm in a hurry and have to just grab something, anything, to eat."

> *Tip: Eat nothing from a bag, a box, or in an individual wrapper.*

Some triggers/ automatic thoughts based on psychology:

- "I'm unsure if this food is really bad for me. Maybe the science is wrong."
- "No one is perfect."
- "I've had a hard day and need some comfort food."
- "I'm sad and tired and don't care what I eat when I feel this way."
- "I deserve to eat what I want."
- "My aunt (uncle, grandparent, parent, sibling, etc.) eats whatever and they are doing fine."

A crucial part of utilizing CBT principles to assist good habit development is to recognize triggers and automatic thoughts. The more you can do this, the easier it will become. Then when a trigger/ automatic thought arises, you can recognize it for

---

[602] Quote attributed to Chef AJ.

what it is and have the CBT tool to think again. You can recognize "stinkin' thinkin'[603] ".

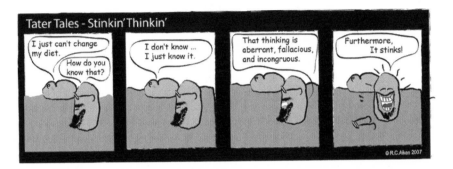

THINK AGAIN

Thoughts inconsistent with your goals, illustrated above, lead to uncomfortable emotions. These emotions may be anger, sadness, apathy, anxiety, or guilt. They cannot be positive emotions because they are against your accepted goals.

When this pattern of trigger, automatic thought with uncomfortable emotion happens, the idea is to "think again."

This process is illustrated below.

---

[603] Quote attributed to co-founder of CBT Albert Ellis.

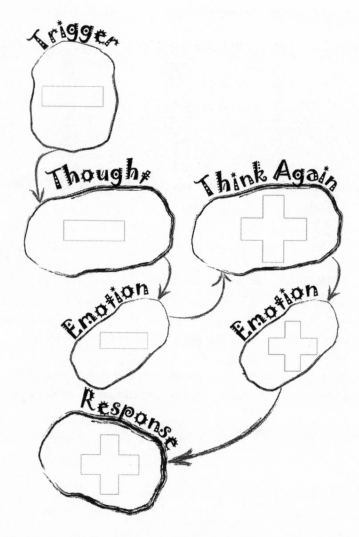

The idea is to think again until the emotion is consistent with your goals. Once the thoughts are more rational, the emotion is more adequate and the behavioral response will be adequate.

It may be of value to formally practice this process until it can be easily accomplished in your head; after a while, a conscious process is unnecessary as triggers no longer affect you. After a time, typical triggers and automatic thinking will become known. To make progress on a deeper psychological level, core beliefs associated with triggers could reveal core beliefs.

If core beliefs are changed, the frequency of situations capable of triggering incongruent thoughts, feelings, and behavior are short-circuited.

THE CBT BRAIN CIRCUIT

Speaking of circuits, there is a very logical medical correlate to the CBT model. Considering the brain as a "processing circuit", first perceptual information is received and "processed" or "analyzed" in the temporal parietal lobe. It is then sent to the second branch, the "emotion circuit," located within the limbic structures, where the initial perception is given emotional meaning. Then the "signal" is sent to the third branch, the "relevance circuit," located in the prefrontal cortex. The response to the emotional content is determined there, whether to use CBT or act out, for example.

This "circuit" can be a handy - if oversimplified - way of understanding the effect of certain emotional disorders on the CBT model. For example psychotic disorders distort perceptions - the first branch of the circuit; affective disorders and anxiety effect the second branch; and behavioral disorders effect the third branch. Corresponding predominant neurotransmitters of these three regions are dopamine, serotonin, and acetylcholine, respectively.

CASE STUDY: STINKIN' THINKIN'

A partner can be very helpful in assisting you with your dietary plan, particularly if that person also adopts the same way of thinking. This is a type of cognitive milieu, which we have detailed in another publication titled *The Cognitive Milieu*[604]. We have also written an accompanying workbook titled *Think Again*[605].

An example follows.

CBT Scene

At home with partner. It's Saturday and you have achieved a lot around the house that day, although not particularly enjoyable tasks. You have been doing fairly well on your whole-food varied-plant diet. Your partner, who has been whole-food varied-plant based for a longer time is supportive. You are hungry and tired.

You: "How about a vegan pizza?"

Partner: "We don't have any – you mean make it from scratch? I've read about pizza with a cauliflower crust?"

You: "No, I mean order to be delivered."

Partner: "There are no vegan pizza deliveries. You don't mean the kind of pizzas we used to order!"

You: "Of course not. Vegetables only."

Partner: "Good luck with ordering whole grain, no salt, no cheese pizza."

---

[604] This book was primarily written for the context of the residential environment for adolescents; R.C. Aiken (2016). *The cognitive milieu.* Go Ahead Publishing, Los Angeles.

[605] This workbook was primarily written for the adolescents and young adults, although its simplicity may be appreciated by older readers; R.C. Aiken (2016). *Think again.* Go Ahead Publishing, Los Angeles.

You: "So what if there is minimal cheese? I'm too tired to make anything and could use a little fun food."

Partner: "That's not fun at all; it's contrary to our principles and our health. You know that. Let me look up the cauliflower recipe and I'll make the best pizza you've ever had. At least best as far as healthy but I think I can make it tasty."

You: "That's really nice of you. Let me help, might be fun."

Analysis

Here the trigger is being tired and automatically thinking that reverting to a previous behavior, although against your current goals, is rationalized. It is distorted thinking that the delivered pizza will in some way closely approximate your chosen diet.

The partner is very important here to point out the fallacy in the proposed delivery and turns the situation into a potentially fun project that expands their dietary choices into a new area of healthy "pizza" with an alternative crust.

DEFENSE MECHANISMS

One type of irrational basis for distorted thinking and resulting irrational behavior is the defense mechanism. Defense mechanisms are defensive behavior adjustments intended to protect oneself from emotional pain. It is important to be aware of the various defense mechanisms and to learn to recognize them and avoid them. Some major types of defense mechanisms follow:

DENIAL

The ability to defend against difficult circumstances and uncomfortable emotions by not recognizing their sources. This defense mechanism is an attempt to refuse to face the facts. Denying the scientific facts behind a whole-food varied-plant diet is an example.

RATIONALIZATION

A conscious effort to defend an action which has produced a feeling of guilt by coming up with a "good reason" for the behavior instead of facing the real reason. Rationalization is a lot like making excuses, except that one really believes the thinking at the time. Making an exception to your diet because of the circumstances is an example.

PROJECTION

Shifting the blame to someone or something else, attributing one's own thoughts or feelings to another. Blaming the environment or the circumstances for not following your diet is an example.

REACTION FORMATION

Reaction formation means to do the opposite of how one feels. An example is while a temporary successful change of eating patterns has been accomplished and is rewarding, one reverts back to the old pattern as if "relapses" are expected and okay.

REGRESSION

Retreating from one's responsibilities in an attempt to return to the comfort of earlier patterns by engaging in those behaviors.

INDEX

A

Acceptable Macro-nutrient
Distribution Range
AMDR, 197
acetylcholine, 204, 365
adaptogenic, 300, 301
adequate Intake
AI, 187, 197, 202, 244
ADHD, ix, 162-163
adolescents, 70- 76, 173, 360, 366, 382
adrenal hormones, 298
adrenal stress, 302
aerobic respiration, **138**
Albert Einstein's son, 34
alchemy, 45
alcohol, 41, 80, 152, 163, 247
alcoholic encephalitis, 50
alkaloids, 162
allergies, 162
almond "milk", 177
alpha brain wave, 275
alpha gal, 175
alpha linolenic acid
ALA, **127**
Alteril, 314-315
Alzheimer's disease, 81, 103, **107**-111, 132, 293
genetic risk, 109
amla, 264
animal fat, 123, 164
anthocyanin, 260, 261, 296
antibacterial, **145**
anticarcinogenic, 298
antidepressant, 39, 122, 126-127, 130, 155, 194, 266-268, 274, 279, 288, 291, 295-296, 302, 309

antidepressants, 104,126-127, 130-131, 190, 266, 268, 289, 294-295
anti-inflammatory, 115-116, 118, 120-123, 134, 145, 148, 150, 155, 194-195, 248, 255-258, 267-268, 272, 278, 288, 295, 298
antimutagenic, 298
antioxidant, xii, xiv, 44, 142, 145,-146, 150, 153-155, 248, 252, 255-257, 261-270, 277, 286, 288, 293, 295-296, 298, 321, 323, 329, 338,-339
anti-psychotic, 104
anxiety, 61, 69-70, 74, 118, 126, 147, 153, 155-156, 165-166, 179, 193, 274-275, 302, 312, 358, 363, 365
anxiolytic, 156, 273, 295
ApoE, 109
apples, 156, 220, 264,337
arachidonic acid, 127, 134, 176, 256
archaea, 303
artichoke, 265
arugula, 252, 346
asafetida, 40
ascorbic acid, 339
ashwagandha, xiii, **301**, 302
aspalathin, 298
asylums, 46, 160
atrial fibrillation, 190
auditory hallucinations, 33, 46
autistic spectrum disorder, 153, 307
autoimmune disorders, 119, 175
automatic thoughts, 361- 362
avocados, 146, 204, 337
Ayurveda, vi, 40, 301
compendia of Caraka, 40

B

B_{12}, 106, 253, 303, 304

Babinski, 98

baking, 258, 259, 270, 281, 319, 322, 334

bananas, 199,204, 264, 337-339, 340

barley, 220, 237

Barnard, 70, 222

Barnes Hospital, 181

basil 269,331, 345, 346

beans, x, 189, 209-210, 220, 263, 278, 280, 286, 323, 327, 329, 344, 351, 353

beet, 144, 146, 252, 253, 346

beetroot, 252-253, 265, 323

behavioral problems, 71, 72

bell peppers, 265, 331, 352

Bernoulli effect, **336**

berries, 260-261, 264, 277, 288, 341, 343, 351

beverages, **263**

Biblical accounts, 41

bidirectional, 158, 159

bioaccessibility, 254, 320-323, 325, 335

bioavailability, 145, 155-156, 252, 290, 335, 344

biohack, 250, 323, 340, 343

bipolar disorder, 105, 125, 129, 130, 152, 181, 193, 204, 279

black beans, 199-200, 209-210, 244, 346-347, 353

black box, 181

black raspberry, 262

black tea, 272

blackberry, 245, 262

Blender Bottle, 343

Blender mechanical properties, **336**

blending, 250, 254, 323-334, 338, 340

blood pressure, 88, 96, 104-105, 110, 181, 234, 243, 246-249, 251- 253, 272, 278, 283, 287, 297, 312

sodium, 105, 178, 181, 244, 246-247, 312, 314

osmosis, 105

blood-brain barrier, 193,204, 287, 315

bloodletting, 89, 160

Bloomindale Insane Asylum, 49

blue green algae, **139**

blueberries, 155, 241, 260-261, 340, 343

blueberries, 264

boiling, 319, 321-334, 336

Book of Daniel, **42**

BPA, 330

Braggs soy sauce, 281

brain, xix, 123

most sensitive organ, 86

second brain, 158

brain death, 86

brain-derived neurotrophic factor, 275

bran, 177-178, 220, 237, 283

Brazil nuts, 266

breakfast, 177, 240-241, 283

Broca, 98

aphasia, 98

broccoli, 129, 146, 199, 227, 244, 312, 321, 323, 330, 341, 343

Bronze Age, **38**

brown rice, 220, 283

Brussels sprouts, 129, 256, 312

Buddha Bowl, 345-346

C

cacao, 245, 258-259, 286

cadmium, 132, 190

caffeine, 273

calcium, 178-179, 219, 306-307, 329

calorie restriction, **213**

Camellia sinensis, 272

carbohydrates, **215**

cardamom, 40

Carl Gustav Jung's mother, 34

carnivores, 303

carotenoids, 122, 146, 150, 186, 252, 295, 320, 329, 335

carrots, 220, 323, 329, 331, 341, 343

catechin, 257

cauliflower, 129, 265,312, 323, 331, 341, 343, 366-367

cavitation, **336**

cayenne, 269

cellulose, 218-219, 329, 335

cerebrovascular disease, vii, xi, **84**, 85, 90-92, 104-106, 116, 232-233
chamomile, 315
Cherokee Plant Medicine teachings, 349
cherry, 262
childhood, 35-36, 70, 75-76, 131
chili, 269
chlorogenic acid, 156
chlorophyll, 122, 320, 329
chlorpromazine, 40
chocolate, 67, 72, 239, 254, 257-259, 262, 270, 286-287, 337
cholecalciferol, 305, 307
cholesterol, vii, 91-93, 95-96, 104, 106, 108-109, 111, 133, 176, 185, 187, 197, 200, 202, 215, 218, 220, 232-240, 277-278, 297, 305, 312, 315
chronic fatigue syndrome, 166
chronic inflammation, 97, 111, 117, 120, 126, 128, 152, 175, 255
chronic pain, **147**
cinnamon, 40, 245, 258, 269
citric acid, 339
clinical death, 85
cloves, 258, 269, 327, 331, 346, 353
Coca-Cola, 263
cocoa, xiii, 257, 285-287
coffee, 156, 241, 245, 263, 279, 337, 351
coffee, 263
Cognitive Behavioral Therapy CBT, xv, 32, **148**,247, 355, 356
cognitive decline, 80-81, 231, 260, 302
cognitive schemata, 357
colectomy, 162
colocynth, 40
Concord grape, 262
consciousness, 28-29, 40, 86
core beliefs, 357-358, 365
cortisol, 148, 279
Cotton, 160
cranberries, 313
creativity, 34, 45, 275
cruciferous, 110, 129, 312, 341, 343
crushing, 88, 235, 310, 323, 344-345

culinary art, 172
cumin, 269
curcumin, 145, 150, 288, 289, 290, 291
curry, 269
cytokines, 117-118, 121, 124, 127,-128, 134, 148, 194, 255

D

dandelions, 150, 269
date syrup, 250, 281
dehydration, 182, 281, 325, 326
delirium, 153, 182
delivery of nutrients, 85
dementia, 50, 79, 80-81, 88, 103-104, 153, 190, 243
demons, 41
denial, xv, 368
DHA, **192**
Dickens, 59
dill, 269
dioxins, 132, 190
docosahexaenoic acid DHA, 68, 127, 187-188, 192-193, 278
dopamine, 120, 203-204, 273, 288, 300, 338, 365
Dream Temples, **39**
dredgers, 245
dutch oven, 353
dysbiosis, 159

E

eating disorders, 153
eggplant, 262,331-332
eicosapentaenoic EPA, 68, 127, 131, 176, 187-188, 193, 278
electroconvulsive therapy, 181
emotion circuit, 365
endothelium, 93, 124, 152, 249, 251
endotoxemia, 123
endotoxin, 124, 255
energy density, xi, 225
enteric nervous system ENS, 158

epithelium, ix, 92, 163
ergocalciferol, 305
erythritol, 258-259
essential amino acids
    EAA, 205, 207-208, 211, 221, 285
Estimated Average Requirement
    EAR, 197
eudaimonia, xix
eukaryotes, 114, 139-140, 218
evolution, 31-32, 36-37, 59, 138, 140,
    141, 159, 201, 221-222, 304
    convergent evolution. *See*
    evolutionary psychiatry, 32
    grains, 282
    Gronk, xx
    balancing selection, 33
exercise, 31, 148, 212, **241**-242, 247,
    250, 253, 297, 302, 356
    Biking, 242
    monitoring, 247, 254

F

farm-raised fish, 189
fermentation, 245, 297
fetal
    development, 77
fiber, 121, 205, 257
fireplace crane, 353
fish liver, 305
flavonoids, 122-123, 252-253, 260-
    261, 278, 296, 338
flavor, xxi, 172-174, 245, 277, 280,
    285, 288, 317, 319-320, 325-326,
    328, 337
    decreased sensation with age, 77
flaxseed, xii, 127, 129, 155, 187-188,
    194, 199-200, 239, 241, 245, 248-
    249, 256, 258-259, 266, 278-281,
    310-312, 343, 346
    wreaths, 282
flourishing, xix
fluoxetine, 289, 294, 309
folic acid, 106, 238, 277
food diary, 315
free radicals, 93, 139, 142, 151, 188,
    259, 322
Freeman, 60

Freezing greens, xiv, 341
Freud, 99
frying, 319, 320, 323

G

gamma-aminobutyric acid, 165
garlic, 40, 44, **233**-234, 239, 245, 281,
    323, 327, 331, 344-346, 353
general paresis of the insane, 51
ginger, 40, 258
Global Burden of Disease study, 276
glucose, 142, 186, 216-218, 283
glucosinolates, 320-321
glycogen, 216
glycolysis, 138, 140, 141
green leafy plants, 333
green peppers, 323, 331
green tea, 155, 239, 250, 255, 257,
    272-273, 274-275, 297
greens, 146, 178, 180, 201, 252, 272,
    341-342, 346, 353
Gronk, v, 25-29, 178
gut luminal endogenous protein, 211
gut-brain axis, **158**

H

headaches, 179, 182
hearth, 350, 352-353
herbal tea, 297, 298
herbicides, 304
herbivores, 303
Hibiscus, xii, xiii, **249**, 250, 296, 297
high speed blender, 327, 333, **337**
high temperature thermal
    processing, **319**
hippocampus, 154-155, 195, 307
Hippocrates, vi, 42, 43, 44, 87, 233
histidine, 205, 210
home garden, 345
Homer's Odyssey, 39
Homo Sapiens
    whole-food varied-plant diet, 27
homocysteine, 106-107, 152
homocysteine hypothesis, 106-107
hops, 315

how to change your dietary pattern, 355
hummus, 282, 327
hygiene hypothesis, 159
hyperforin, 150
hyperthyroidism, 312
hypothalamic-pituitary-adrenal HPA, 147, 274
hypothalamus, 268, 301, 307
Hypothyroidism, 312

I

imipramine, 162, 266, 268, 294
immune, 123
immune system, 76, 113-114, 116-117, 119, 127, 151, 159, 161
Inflammation, **254**
inflammatory biomarkers, 122, 124, 133
inflammatory response., 111, 148
innate immune system, 113-114, 118
insanity, 32, 33, 40-41, 46-47, 100, 160
insomnia, 179, 299, 302
interferon, 124-125
Intestinal permeability, 163
iodine, **311**, 312, 313, 314
    iodine deficiency, 312
Iodine deficiency, 311
isoleucine, 205, 210

J

James Joyce's daughter, 34
jejube, 40
junk foods, **71**

K

kale, 146, 199, 201, 227, 244, 256, 265, 272, 326-327, 334-345
kernels, 260
King George III, 49
kiwis, 204
Kraepelin, 100

L

Lactobacillus, 165-167
lacto-ovo vegetarians, 189, 208
lanolin, 305
lead, 28-29, 32, 35, 37, 78, 85, 91, 106, 111, 132, 135, 143, 148, 152, 159, 176, 181, 187, 190, 220, 233, 243, 309, 312, 357, 361, 363
leafy greens, 121, 201
leafy vegetables, xii, 110, 252, 272, 320, 333, 341-342, 344
leaky gut, ix, 164
legal death, 85
legumes, 65, 120, 191, 209-210, 227, 257, 278
lemon, 180, 250, 264, 327, 339, 342, 346, 353
leucine, 205, 210
lichen, 305, 310
lignan, 248, 255, 279
lime, 180, 250, 264, 339-340, 342
lipids, 108, 110, 185, 235, 238, 239, 283
lipophilic, 320-321, 322
lithium, 178, 180-182
low-density lipoproteins, 111
lower temperature thermal processing, **323**
L-theanine, 273-274
lysine, 205, 209-210

M

Maca, xiii, 289, 300-301
macronutrients, 133, 174, 183, 185, 198, 215-216, 221, 334
mad as a hatter, 47
magnesium, 177-180, 207, 238, 277, 283, 329
maniacs, 49
meat, 26-27, 29, 42, 61-65, 68-69, 80, 106, 109-110, 116, 122-123, 133-134, 164, 175, 189, 198, 207, 264, 270, 320
Mediterranean Diet, 64-67, 80, 110, 121
megavitamin therapy, 145

melancholia, 46
melatonin, 315
mental disorders
    earliest evidence, 38
    genetic susceptibility, 35
mental Disorders
    beginning, 27
mental effort, 217
mercury, 45, 47, 132, 190, 192
methionine, 106, 205, 210
microbiome, 157-158, 165, 167, 219
microorganisms, 157-159, 163, 320
microwave, 241, 319
mild cognitive impairment, 79
mind-body-spirit, 99
mint, 256, 269, 341, 352
mitochondrion, 138, 156
    mitochondrial disorder, 156
molybdenum catalysis, 306
monoamine oxidase inhibition, 300
monoamine theory of depression,
    203
monounsaturated fatty acids, 238
mood disorders
    prevalence, 53
    relatively recent phenomenon, 59
mortar and pestle, 334, 344

neurogenesis, x, 155, 195, 289
neuroimmune, 158
neuroinflammation, 134, 176, 192
neurologic development, 76
neuroprotection, 194
neuroprotective, 110, 182, 275, 278,
    287, 293, 298
neuroregeneration, 154
neurotoxicity, 106
neurotransmitter, 102, 120, 194, 203,
    275
New York Hospital, 49
niacin, 175, 285
nitrate, 251-253
nitrates, 252, 272
nitric oxide, 249, 251-252, 254, 297
nitrogen, 151, 205, 208, 212-213, 303
non-steroidal anti-inflammatories,
    163, 289
norepinephrine, 120, 204
nothofagin, 298
NSAIDs, 246
nutmeg, 269
nutraceuticals, 288, 290
nutraceutics, 288, 343
nutrient density, xi, 176, 225-228
nutritional yeast, xii,285, 327, 345

N

National Academies Institute of
    Medicine, 305
National Academies Press, 186-188,
    197, 200, 219, 232, 312
National Comorbidity Survey, 52, 71,
    76
National Institute of Mental Health,
    xix, 126, 164
Nepenthe, 39
Nepenthes pharmakon, 39
Neu5Gc, 175
neural tissue, 117
neurobiological, 116, 147-148
neurodegeneration, 110, 117, 151
neurodegenerative, 106-107, 117,
    254, 273-275, 293, 302, 338
neuroendocrine, 158
neurogastronomy, ix, 172

O

oat flour, 258, 259
oatmeal, 241, 256, 280
oats, 178, 220, 237, 241, 258, 283
obesity, 71, 75, 96, 125, 147, 163,
    220, 247, 254, 287
obsessive compulsive disorder, 274
Okinawa traditional diet, xi, 223
old friends theory, 159
omega-3, x, 68, 121, 127-132, 155,
    186-188, 191-192, 194-197, 199-
    202, 256, 272, 278-280, 310, 347
omega-3 supplements, 310
omega-6, 121, 127-128, 134, 176,
    194-197, 199-202, 278, 347
omnivores, 68-70, 115, 134
onion, 234, 281, 323, 331-332
onions, 234, 323, 344, 352, 353
oregano, 269, 331

organochlorine pesticides, 190
osteomalacia, 306
oxidation, 337
oxidative stress, viii, 76, 106, 109,
    121, 135, 137, 139, 142, 148, 151-
    153, 259, 277, 283, 287
oxygen radical, 117

P

Paleolithic Period
    Gronk, 25
    middle, 25
    scavenging, 27
panic disorder, 274
parsley, 256
passionflower, 315
pastes, 326, 345
pathogens, 113, 117-118, 148, 151,
    285
Pauling, 145
peanuts, 256, 265-266
peas, 204, 278, 330
pecans, 238, 241, 256, 277
pellicle, 265-266
pepper, 40, 145, 265, 269, 290-291,
    327, 331-332, 343, 346, 353
persistent organic pollutants
    POPs, 132, 190
pesco vegetarian, 208
pesticides, 303
pestos, 345
pharmaceutics, 190, 288, 294
phenolic, 150, 278, 337-338
phenolic acids, 278
phenylalanine, 205, 210, 338
photosynthesis, 122, 140-141, 177,
    185, 205, 216
phthalates, 330
Physicians Committee for
    Responsible Medicine, 222
physiological stress, 213
phytochemicals, 146, 153, 253, 256,
    270, 292, 320
phytonutrient, 228, 252, 288
phytonutrients, 42, 116, 145, 216,
    219, 226, 283, 301, 329, 334, 338-
    339, 347

phytoplanktonic algae, 305
phytosterols, 133
pineapples, 204
Pinel, 32
piperine, 145, 289-291
pistachios, 256, 266
pituitary, 147, 268, 274, 301
plant stanols, 235-236, 238-240, 277
plasticizers, 330
plums, 156, 204, 260, 262
polybrominated diphenyl ethers, 190
polychlorinated biphenyls
    PCBs, 132, 190
polyphenolesterase, 321, 337
polyphenols, 141, 155-156, 219, 249,
    250, 254-256, 273-274, 279, 287,
    297-298, 320-321, 329, 338, 340
polyunsaturated fatty acids
    PUFAs, 121, 128, 131, 163, 186,
    189, 256
pomegranate, 40, 279
portfolio diet, 239-240, 280, 315
post-partum depression, 129
post-traumatic stress disorder, 125,
    154
potatoes, 64, 133, 312-313, 330, 344,
    352-353
predator-prey, 138
Premenstrual Syndrome, 295
primate, 129, 174, 200, 334
probiotics, 165-166
processed foods, 72-74, 84, 121, 123,
    198, 245, 312
processing circuit, 365
projection, xv, 368
prokaryote, 303
prostaglandins, 246
protein, **203**
provitamin D_2, 305
psychiatrists, 33, 60, 65, 98-99, 161
psychoanalytic, 99, 160
psychobiotics, **164,** 166
psychological stress, 31, 147-148,
    152, 163, 247
    beginning of mental disorders, 31
psychosis, 47, 107, 156, 162, 179
psychosocial stress, 135
psychosocial stressor, 125

psychosurgery, 161
psychotropic, 100, 165, 166, 181, 288
PUFAs, **127**
pumpkin seeds, 256
pyridoxine, 106

Q

quinone, 339

R

radish, 40
raspberries, 264
rational, 28, 32, 45, 177, 364
rationalization, xv, 368
Rauvolfia serpentina, 40
reaction Formation, xv, 368
recipe
    anti-inflammatory brownies, 258
    Flax Craxs, 279
    Sous vide ratatouille Nicoise, 331
    super smoothie, 342
    Hibiscus and green tea workout
        drink, 250
    Kale yes chips, 325
    Portfolio overnight oatmeal
        breakfast, **240**
    smoothie recipe for health and
        happiness, 339
    Stone Age Buddha bowl, 345
Recommended Dietary Allowance
    RDA, 197, 202
Red Bull energy drink, 263
red cabbage, 265
red raspberry, 262
reductionist approach, 144, 145, 228
regression, xv, 369
Reil, 50
    psychiaterie, 50
relevance circuit, 365
resistant starch, 121, 219
Rett's disorder, 153
rhizobia, 303
rhodiola, xiii, 289, 299-301
riboflavin, 175, 285
rickets, 306
right angle mixture

RAM, 224
roasting, 263, 319, 334
roasting and cooking over an open
    fire, 349
Rooibos, **297**
Rudyard Kipling, xx

S

sacred disease, 86
sacred four-directions harvest table
    vegan thanksgiving, **349**
saffron, xiii, **267**-269, 291-293, 295
safranal, 295
sage, 258, 269, 352
salicylic acid, 114-116
salt, vii, xii, 55, 105, 181, 244-245,
    312, 366
sandalwood, 40
satiation, 220, 343
saturated fat, vii, 111, 176, 202
schizophrenia, 32-35, 116, 125, 152,
    154, 195, 204, 274, 307
schizotypal personality disorder, 34
sea salt, 312
seasonal affective disorder, 129, 308
seaweed, 313
secondary metabolites, 60, 288
serotonin, 36, 102, 120, 203-204,
    273, 288, 291, 295, 300, 365
serotonin pathway, 102
sertraline, 266
sickness behavior, 118
sip and swirl, 343
sleep, 125, 148, 153, 217, 314, 315
sleep supplements, xiii, 314
smell, 172-174, 280
    orthonasal smell, 172
    retronasal smell, 173
smoking, 80, 96, 125, 247
smoothie, 201, 297, 333, 340-343
Socratic questioning, 359
solar energy cells, 151
soluble fiber, **237**
sourdough bread, 352, 353
sous vide, xiv, **328**-330
soy powder, 241
Soy protein, **236**

spinach, 146, 178, 204, 252, 256, 265, 312, 323
spouted wheat, 244
sprouted, 345, 346

ß

ß-glucans, 237

S

St. John's wort, 150, **266**, 269
Standard American Diet
SAD, 198, 200, 223
starches, 216, 219
statins, 315
steaming, 319, 321
stinkin' thinkin', 363
Stone Age, xiv, 25-26, 283, 344-345
strawberries, 150, 260, 340, 343
stroke
depression, 101
emotional, behavioral, and cognitive decline, 101
hemorrhagic stroke, 88, 91, 104, 243
high blood pressure, 105
hyperintensities, 105
injury caused by any disruption of blood supply, 88
ischemic stroke. See
micro-strokes, 97
mini-stroke, 97
personality changes, 101
silent stroke, 102
struck down by unknown force, 88
subtle and gradual in effect, 102
thrombosis, 90, 106
suicide, 35, 41, 46, 65, 77, 117, 179, 180, 191-192, 196
sun's energy, 259, 333
supplements, **302**
Plant stanols, sterols, xiii, 315
sweet potato, 265
symbiosis, 138, 158, 305
sympathetic nervous system, 147, 148

synaptic plasticity, 194, 195
synergy, viii, 143-146

T

Taiyo Kagaku Company of Japan, 276
Talmud, 41
taste, 42-43, 166, 172-174, 250, 277, 280, 287-288, 291, 332-334, 337, 353, 361
bitter, 42-43, 150, 172-174, 202, 250, 264-265, 277, 280, 334-335, 343
sweet, 42, 75, 172-174, 199, 265, 277, 312, 334, 343-344
TATER, 360
texture, 173, 280, 320, 325, 341, 344, 346
Thanksgiving, 349, 352
The Cognitive Milieu, 366, 382
The New Ancestral Diet, xvii, 27, 96, 174, 221-222, 334, 382
theanine, 273-276, *See* L-theanine
thiamine, 175, 285
Think again, xv, xxi, 360, 363, 366, 382
Thorazine, 40, 162, 181
threonine, 205, 210
thyme, 258, 331
tomatoes, 110, 146, 199, 204, 227, 331-332, 351, 353
toxicity, 42, 181, 306
toxins, 113, 118, 123, 152, 161, 163, 188
trans-fat, 176, 198, 202
tree nuts, 133, 237, 239-241, 256, 277
trepanation, **38**
triggers, 93, 98, 134, 148, 361-362, 364
triglycerides, 106, 109, 186
trivet, 352
tryptophan, 203, 205, 210, 315
Tuke, 47
turmeric, 40, 145, 150, 245, 258, 269, 288-290, 291, 327, 343, 346
tyrosine, 203, 338

U

underground storage organs
USOs, 227, 344
UVB, 304-305

V

valerian, 40, 315
valine, 205, 210
vascular disease, 44, 83, 90, 103,
108,-109, 117, 119, 128, 132, 142,
147, 150, 152, 176, 196, 223, 232,
233-234, 243, 259, 277, 283, 287
atherosclerotic plaques, 108
vegan, 70, 239, 313
vegetable wash solution, 342
vegetarian diet, 66, 68-69, 134
vertical garden, 345
Virchow, 90
vitamin A, 175
vitamin B_{12}, 291, 303
vitamin C, 141-142, 145-146, 153-
154, 175, 329, 339
vitamin D, 125, 224, **304**-310
vitamin D_2, 305, 310
vitamin D_3, 305, 307, 310
Vitamix Turboblend VS, 342

W

walnuts, 121, 127, 199, 200, 238,
241, 256, 258, 265-266, 277, 327,
345, 350-351

Washington University in St. Louis,
180, 382
water, 85, 105, 138, 140, 149-150,
177-178, 181-182, 190, 199, 205,
212, 218-220, 243, 250-251, 263,
281, 297, 298, 303, 320, 321, 323,
325, 327-328, 332-333, 338, 341-
343, 346
watercress, 256
whole grain, xiii, 121, 282-283
wild blueberry, 262
wild-caught fish, 189
window of anabolic opportunity, 212
wine, 263
Winokur, 180
World Health Organization, xx, 53,
54, 219

X

xenohormesis, **149**

Y

yarrow, 269

Z

zombie, 25
zucchini, 323, 331-332, 341, 343

AUTHOR

Richard Aiken holds a PhD from Princeton University and an MD from the University of Utah, where he also was a tenured professor. His adult residency and child fellowship were at Washington University in St. Louis. He is a board-certified psychiatrist.

He has written numerous articles in peer-reviewed journals and books. His most recent books are the *Think Again* cognitive behavioral workbook for adolescents and young adults, *The Cognitive Milieu* for residential treatment of adolescents, and *The New Ancestral Diet* detailing why "Paleo" is actually vegan.

Dr. Aiken taught and researched at the Eidgenössische Technische Hochschule in Zürich, Switzerland, as well as the Kungliga Tekniska Högskolan in Stockholm, Sweden. He has lectured throughout the United States, Europe, and in the Middle East.

Dr. Aiken encourages contact:

email: rcaiken@alumni.Princeton.edu
website: www.moodforlife.com
social: Twitter @rcaiken

Made in the USA
Middletown, DE
21 February 2020